Life...
or Grave Danger?

To my dear friend Bob

Wishing you the best in happiness,
health + prosperity;

Blessing,

[signature]   Nov/2013

Life...
or Grave Danger?

Life...
or Grave Danger?

Doug Widdifield

*"It is the nature of humankind to be healthy…
God made no errors when he created man and woman…"*

Life...or Grave Danger?

A Brijess Publication

Printed in the United States of America

Copyright 2013 – Doug Widdifield - Brijess Holdings, Inc.

All rights reserved.

Brijess Publishing

Brijess Holdings, Inc., 2019 Bobtail Circle

Henderson, NV 89012

702.363.0272

Hard Copy Version

ISBN 978-0-615-85783-1

Widdifield, Doug

Life… Or Grave Danger?

Cover & Interior Design by: Dianne Leonetti - DzinerGraphics.com

Testimonials

"My relationship with Doug Widdifield spans over 20 years. I have lectured with him and accompanied him to China in 1999 where we addressed the Chinese Ministry of Health and various dignitaries in parliament. This book is changing lives! It is destined to become a classic."

–Dr. Herbert DeloRey - Board Certified Naturopath
Featured in the book *Great Minds of the 21ˢᵗ Century*

ഏരദ

"Doug and I have collaborated and lectured on health together since the late 1980s and have enjoyed a mutual kinship over the years. His book is a very enlightening and commonsensical approach to the body's functionality and its relation to a healthy lifestyle and health care. A must read for everyone!"

–Dr. Arthur Davis Jr. M.D.

ഏരദ

"Doug has taken the complex subject of nutrition that many doctors have had no, none, zero, zip, nada training in and put it into terms that are easy to read, understand and apply. If you want to take control of your health instead of leaving it to someone else—this is the book for you. By applying the basic principles that Doug teaches in this book, you and your family can enjoy a much healthier life and avoid the vast majority of the degenerative diseases associated with aging.

Today many are in business to make as much money as fast as they can—even if it means cutting corners with your health. Don't believe it? The reason their so-called "foods" have such a long shelf life is because they put damaging chemical preservatives in it, expose it to radiation, and/ or produce modified genetics that can't digest efficiently and the bugs can't live on it. That being reality, their so called "foods" will also cause your body to become sick and eventually die. It simply takes longer because your body is much bigger—and many of these things are cumulative— meaning they concentrate in your body tissues over time.

Still aren't convinced? Buy a tomato in the market and pick one fresh from the garden. The market tomato tastes like cardboard while the garden tomato is bursting with flavor. Based upon Doug's years of nutritional experience in the animal industry in Canada and additional years of research in providing nutrient rich products for the human and animal families—he helps you understand why there is such a dramatic difference between actual foods and "fake foods".

As a physician I have collaborated with Doug for several years and have developed a definite respect for his knowledge. I am confident that you will feel the same way after reading this book."

–C.C. Wilcher, D.C., N.M.D., C.Ac., D.N.B.H.E., D.I.A.M.A
Author of the book–*The Universal Laws of Healing*

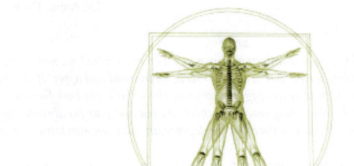

Table of Contents

Dedication

DR. LEO V. ROY, B.A., M.D., N.D., F.A.N.A.

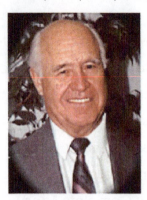

Dr. Roy practiced as a family doctor for seven years as well as having over 35 years of training and experience in natural health care and preventative medicine.

Besides being house physician at Dr. Max Gerson Cancer Clinic in New York, Dr. Roy was a visiting physician to health clinics and centers of natural methods of research in Europe, Asia and throughout North America. He was a longtime friend and mentor to me and travelled in concert with me—sharing his wisdom, love and knowledge with the people of North America and Asia.

Dr. Roy's naturopathic approach to healing—fought disease by caring for and restoring the total health of the body, mind, emotions and spirit.

He taught me that healing is not a casual pastime nor is it a spectator sport. He believed that everything in your life…your home, your loved ones, your friends and your successes—depends upon your state of health, your inner and personal life, your emotions and your happiness.

Dr. Roy's pearls of wisdom:
"You are all you have.
Look after yourself well.
Keep joy in your life!"

I dedicate this book in his memory. – Doug Widdifield

Acknowledgements

First and foremost, I would like to acknowledge my fabulous wife, Krystyna, for all her support and assistance in bringing this project to reality. Without her relentless effort, long hours and belief, this book would have been no more than a wishful dream fading with time. Thank you sweetheart!

I also want to acknowledge my late mentor–Dr. Leo Roy. He is as much, and possibly even more, the real author of this manuscript. It was Dr. Roy that taught me the philosophy of letting complete whole foods and/or complete whole food supplements be our medicine. It was also Dr. Roy that first taught me that virtually all degenerative conditions are the result of poisons and toxins rather than viruses, germs and bacteria–as we have been taught and conditioned to believe.

I would also like to recognize the continued support of my recently deceased friend Dr. Arthur Davis Jr. M.D. He blessed me with his friendship and support for almost a quarter of a century–and will be very much missed.

Currently, I am humbled to have such brilliant healers as Dr. Charles Wilcher (author of *The Universal Laws Of Healing*) and Dr. Herbert DeloRey as both wonderful friends, colleagues and mentors. They have also contributed greatly to making this book possible and I am truly grateful.

I would also like to give thanks to my dear friends Dennis Richard (author of *Your Health Is Your Choice*) and Mark Matulis for their participation and support.

I want to acknowledge Carol Adler (Dandilion Books) for all she has done in editing, writing and arranging all the material into a readable format. Also Dianne Leonetti (D'ziner Graphics) for all the illustrations, graphic design and print setting necessary for completion.

I also want to acknowledge and thank many others that made significant contributions to this project–it would be virtually impossible to name them all. Last, but certainly not least, I want to give thanks to my Creator–for His guidance.

Author's Note

In order to absorb and best utilize all of the information contained in this book, I suggest the following procedure:

1. Read through the entire book, from start to finish.
2. Choose the chapters that seem to apply most directly to you and your health questions or challenges.
3. Reread and study those chapters. Take notes.
4. Read through the entire book once again, this time more carefully. Take notes on the other chapters that were not on your priority list.

By using this process you will soon discover the following:

1. Instead of providing summaries at the end of each chapter, the entire book is a map or journey that starts at the point of presenting the problem and then delivers the solution.
2. When you follow this problem-solving wellness-based journey through the book you will find much of the information repeated where it needs to be applied to specific areas that are covered in that chapter.
3. The 4 principles of wellness presented in Chapter 1 will be emphasized many times throughout the book.
4. If you learn and apply those 4 principles, you will have taken a major step—a leap—in the direction of improving the quality of your life, day by day, in so many ways.

You will note that I have used the masculine gender throughout the book when referring to both male and female genders. Please understand this is merely to make it easier to read, instead of bogging down the reader with "her or she" or "him or her" every time a gender issue occurs.

In some instances product or trade names of specific healing herbs or formulas are mentioned, since there is no other way to refer to them. I have included these herbal products because I believe they have such high healing capabilities, they deserve to appear in any book that provides the latest comprehensive information about wellness and healing.

—*Douglas Widdifield*

Preface

The title of this book, *Life…or Grave Danger?* includes a play on words. It asks you, the reader to make a choice between "living" or "grave dying"—"grave" as in "serious," and "grave" as in the kind that exists in a cemetery.

Both adjective and noun definitions of "grave" have the same implication. We can have a healthy, robust life experience that is exciting and productive; or a boring, lackluster one that is mere "existence"—low energy, poor health and nothing to look forward to except survival from the last head cold, flu or surgery. We all know people whose only excitement or adventure in life is their last operation.

Everything in life is a choice, our choice. Who we are and what we become is for the most part a result of the choices we make, whether consciously or subconsciously. We make those choices based on available information, unconscious programming, experience, observation, and conscious decisions to question the known and explore the unknown.

We derive logical and intelligent choices from truthful or validated information— tested facts, recorded observation, and personal experience. Surely no one wants to keep making the same choices if they only continue to lead to unhappy, unproductive or unhealthy outcomes.

Poor choices are generally the result of perverted, skewed or inaccurate information. Information that is deliberately skewed is called propaganda. Propaganda is one of the best ways to control the beliefs, habits and resources of a nation or society.

If you believe, for example, that "things go better with Coke" (a 1963 Coca Cola slogan), or that Coke really is "the pause that refreshes" (a 1929 Coca Cola slogan)… or that Coke is "the real thing" (a 1970s Coca Cola slogan) then you will reach for a coke or cola drink whenever you're looking for a refreshing, energizing, authentic, *GREAT feeling about life*: that refreshing feeling, or that feeling of being "in" with the "real" crowd, the "right" crowd—the people who "really matter."

In 1971, Coca Cola charmed the world with a multi-media ad campaign and slogan, "I'd like to buy the world a coke," subconsciously linking Coca Cola with world unity, peace, fun and laughter throughout the world (even in countries where people are starving and have NO food, let alone nutritious food). With a Coca Cola bottle in hand and black, white, yellow, brown and red people dancing and singing, the whole world looks brighter and peace is right around the corner—yes? It kind of goes with blue jeans, a bright (cavity-free) smile, the right car, job and boy or girlfriend. By now ("buy now"—another subconscious programming phrase often used in sales campaigns), most of the educated, informed and aware community knows that the ingredients in Coca Cola can easily dissolve rusty nails and clean out clogged drain pipes. This sugary roto-rooter synthetic drink wreaks havoc in the body. Too much coke can not only lead to sugar highs, sugar blues, weight gain, and diabetes… it can also lead a person down the road of other junk food habits and a matching lifestyle.

Yet, how many of these educated, enlightened individuals continue to reach for a coke and drink it or one of its cola/soft drink derivatives over quality bottled water or fresh-squeezed juice?

Because of this heavy subconscious programming, when it comes to health and healing—life and death matters—our discernment, even our common sense often takes a back seat to fear-based propaganda. The program running in our minds is: *"What if we make the "wrong" choices… choices that go against almost everything the hospital, drug and medical industries tell us is the "right" way to stay healthy and fit?"*

What if we know without a doubt that certain medical claims or procedures are false, misleading and even dangerous? Our subconscious programming then takes over with the following script: *"Yet the other way, the alternative route, could be just as false and misleading. Therefore, isn't it better to go along with what the government, its agencies and their authorities advise and promote? Anyway, we have health insurance that pays most of those costs. It makes sense."*

Whenever fear sets in, our self-confidence slinks into a corner. Programming can be powerful. We know what happened to Galileo when he claimed the sun did not revolve around the earth. Likewise, we know what happens today to health practitioners and researchers who come up with non-invasive (drug and surgery-free) permanent solutions to health challenges.

Bottom Line: Today we live in a heavily regulated society that tries to make most of our health choices for us. Many of us are no longer willing to offer ourselves as sacrifices on the altars of a medical science controlled by plutocrats and big industry.

In the food arena, likewise, the Food and Drug Administration determines and rules for or against "healthy food choices" and "questionable," "quack" or "placebo" food supplements.

In this book you will find information about disease, including cancer and other serious health challenges that medical doctors do not generally share with their patients. You will also find information that may be new or that contradicts what you believe to be true about optimal health and health care.

This book dispels some of the most popular myths about food and food supplements.

I invite you to read its contents with an open mind and to evaluate its validity, accuracy and truthfulness to determine if it resonates with your philosophy.

"It is the nature of humankind to be healthy...
God made no errors when he created man and woman..."

Chapter 1

How Do We Know What's Good For Us?

We have to be good detectives and astute researchers in order to make sure we're making the right food and other health choices.

As North Americans in many ways we're fortunate because we have such a plentiful supply of food to choose from. The flip side of the coin is the challenge of making the right choices. Competition can be overwhelming.

The easy way out is to rely on authority—the experts. As mentioned in the Preface, we don't have to go far to be told where to find those authorities. In fact, our society is set up to make most of our decisions for us.

We also discussed the pitfalls of allowing the marketplace to determine our choices. For example, fast food is convenient, low cost, available, and reliable. We know what to expect from any of the hamburger, burrito or fried chicken franchises, whether in Laramie, Wyoming; Plattsburg, New York; or Lake Charles, Louisiana. When analyzing nutritional value, most of us have learned by now that most fast food falls far short of the quality nutrition our bodies seek in order to maintain optimal health. Most of it can be classified as junk food because its ingredients are highly toxic, denatured, over-processed and often rancid.

Would it not be better to make our own choices? To do our own research by observing, asking questions, reading extensively, consulting with a number of individuals who support different philosophies and perspectives—and finally, test different foods and brands ourselves, to learn if they agree with our specific body systems? Of course.

We have to be good detectives and astute researchers in order to be assured of making the right food and other health choices specifically for our body type. Also, we must keep up with the latest information regarding nutritional supplements. Even though we may be motivated to make healthy choices, we are constantly confronted with misinformation. Truthful information can easily be skewed to become misleading.

How crucial is it to spend time educating ourselves about nutrition? We can answer that question with another: *Is anything more important than our health?*

It is a fact that "we are what we eat," whether eating refers to the consumption of nutritional food, "empty" or non-nutritional food, information, disinformation, propaganda, enriching and uplifting experiences, or empty, depressing ones.

Which do YOU prefer—disease care or health care?

Often people become confused about the difference between health care and disease care. Logically, if we consider ourselves healthy and whole, we will live accordingly and make healthy, wholesome lifestyle choices. Our calendar will not be cluttered with doctors' appointments and tests in order to make sure nothing's wrong. If we have a headache, for example, our common sense will tell us we're tired, we need to slow down or some issue is troubling us that needs our attention. A headache does not necessarily mean onset of flu or a cold, a tumor somewhere, or the need to consider having our gall bladder removed!

Disease Care

Conventional medicine, often called Western or allopathic medicine, is based on a disease model for diagnosis and treatment.[1] When a person visits an allopathic doctor, they subject themselves to an examination of their physical bodies, just as one would take a vehicle to an auto repair shop to determine if all the parts are working well or if one or more of them need fixing.

All vehicles that are the same style, make and year are treated alike. Likewise, all individuals who fit certain categories on the medical charts (age, sex, height and weight, etc.) are treated objectively, as physical "machines" or mechanisms. The doctor will diagnose, based on the guidelines stated on the chart or in the database. He will also determine which medicines to prescribe, based on a pharmaceutical reference book, the PDR or *Physicians' Desk Reference*®. Statistics or predictable patterns (aka labels) are a doctor's and auto mechanic's best friends.

The premise upon entering the doctor's office is that something may be wrong, even if the patient is experiencing no pain or presenting other symptoms. In other words, the patient asks the doctor to *confirm* that nothing's wrong with him. Essentially

---

1. Conventional Western medicine [or allopathic medicine], is organized around the Theory of Diseases, which believes that a person becomes sick because he or she contracts a disease. In this model, each disease is seen as an independent entity which can be fully understood without regard to the person it afflicts or the environment in which it occurs. Conventional treatments are treatments of diseases, not of people. Most of the drugs employed in conventional medicine are designed to act as chemical strait jackets, preventing the cells of the body from performing some function that has become hyperactive. – Dr. Jon Cat, http://curezone.com/art/read.asp?ID=161&db=1&C0=13
The Conventional approach to the treatment of most illnesses, mild or serious, is routinely to hit the condition with drugs or surgery. Here again is a quick-fix even though imminent death is not being averted and drugs in particular that are designed to attack one set of symptoms invariably cause problems and malfunctions in other areas of the body. Conventional medicine's approach is to treat symptoms, not the underlying causes. from the arteries. Very little is done to investigate and discover and understand the reason WHY, for that individual, cholesterol is rising. http://www.medicineinformation.info/conventional-medicine-vs-alternative-medicine.html

the patient gives the doctor full responsibility for examining him, i.e., to search for symptoms of disease, even when the patient has no reason to believe otherwise.

For the allopathic doctor, symptoms are signals that one or more body parts needs fixing. Treatment or repair is performed by antidotes to relieve the presenting symptoms: an aspirin for a headache or an antibiotic for a cold or the flu, and surgery for mending or replacing a malfunctioning body part.

It is a well-known fact that allopathic medicine is designed and targeted to treat only symptoms. In no way does it promote the healing of degenerative or chronic conditions. As a matter of fact, this form of medicine seldom if ever addresses the causes of these conditions. They are generally left untouched and unknown. Medical doctors have no solutions for a person who is physically well but feeling depressed, tired, often angry and resentful, weak and exhausted.

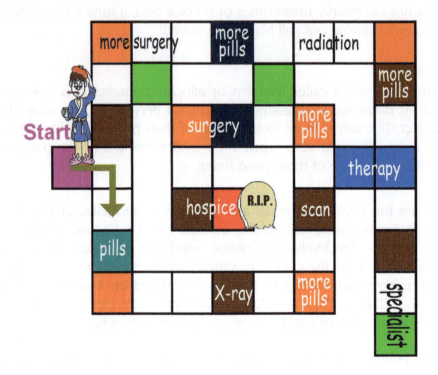

Consider the benefits of promoting disease care as health care, i.e., to focus on treating symptoms rather than addressing causes of specific health challenges. The end result is a patient who keeps coming back for more treatments and more medications.

Treating symptoms can never lead to discovery and treatment of causes. From a marketing standpoint, any business is profitable if it develops a large database of returning customers. The disease care industry is profit motivated to keep patients from recovering from their diagnosed disease or illness and creating a dependency on prescription medication.

The questions often unvoiced by people who subscribe to the conventional medical model are: *Can we ever be well or free from problems? Is life merely a downhill journey to death? Is there a lifestyle or roadmap other than the one that leads people through routine checkups, tests and more tests, visits to one specialist after another, inevitable surgery with accompanying drugs until they end up in assisted living facilities, nursing homes, hospices, and finally the cemetery?*

The answer to this question is, yes. There certainly is another path everyone can take if they choose.

Health care – the truth about healing

It is the nature of humankind to be healthy. God made no errors when He created man and woman.

Balance is essential to wellness. Everything in nature is a struggle for balance. Imbalance creates complications and chaos. It is only when we violate Nature's laws via excesses, abuses and harmful mind-sets that we attract disease and imbalance in our lives.

In order to overcome the challenges of body imbalances, we must first understand and address these violations. Only then, can we remove all healing barriers that prevent us from enjoying the wellness that was designed for us by our Creator.

The first step in healing is to understand and accept that disease is really nothing more than "dis-ease"—a condition of being ill at ease or uncomfortable. Dis-ease is merely a body that is out of balance. It follows that if we can assist in bringing the body back to a state of balance, we can eliminate the dis-ease.

If this is correct, then it would logically follow that "balance" in the body is the magic bullet that science and researchers have been seeking since the beginning of time.

Balance = Wellness

Healthy living and enjoyment of life require emotional balance, physical and structural balance, balance between work and play, and balanced habits and mindsets. Lack of perfect balance in the entire body creates health challenges and blocks the body's ingenious attempts to restore health.

Body balancing (healing) can be as complex as is the nature of the challenge. Chronic and degenerative diseases are extremely complex. Determining their nature and their curing require both consideration and understanding. Healing or curing a significant health challenge requires that we first find and understand all the causes and then eradicate these causes.

By removing an unhealthy organ or tumor by surgery or destroying it by radiation, we fail to discover and address what caused that organ to become unhealthy in the first place.

Curing does not occur by merely relieving symptoms and distresses. Curing does occur if we eliminate the cause(s) and restore the whole body to its optimum well-being.

Cutting, burning and drugging may relieve some of the presenting symptoms, such as pain, lethargy, and indigestion, but this relief is only superficial. It is merely a band-aid that does not address the problem itself.

Any sign of pain or other symptoms are a message that some area of the body is out of balance. To bring the body into balance or *homeostasis*, a wellness-oriented health practitioner will *search for the cause of the imbalance or weakness and treat that causal factor.* Treatment is a personal matter. The patient is not a statistic nor can the treatment and care of their body follow a pre-formulated recipe.

Nature, including human nature, is a tyrant. It strives for and demands perfection. Those who listen to and respect Nature's demands are nobly rewarded. Nature exacts a serious toll for those who refuse to listen.

The human body, mind and emotions are almost infinite in scope and complexity. Possibly several hundred thousand biochemical reactions normally occur in the body metabolism. Hundreds of thousands of things could go wrong and cause disease. Consider the enormous number of possible structural, glandular and emotional imbalances and disharmonies that can occur between the values and principles by which people live, and the needs of their real nature.

The body systems contain hundreds of thousands of enzymes, hundreds of minerals and over 50 vitamins. Each of these can be deficient, excessive, toxic, out of balance with others, or with the body itself.

FOUR BASIC PRINCIPLES OF OPTIMAL HEALTH

Following are the 4 principles that are the foundation for achieving and maintaining optimal health:

1. **The body systems must be clean in order to function optimally**

   Have you ever started to light a fire over a mound of cold ashes? Or move brand new household furnishings into a mold-and-mildew, roach-infested home, or one with dirty carpets, dirty walls, piles of trash in the corners of the room? Or, did you ever try to hike on a path that is cluttered with rocks, fallen tree limbs and debris?

In order for any solid or liquid nutrient to provide full value, the body must be clean. The "ducts" or capillaries and arteries must be open without any blockage that would impede the free flow of oxygen, water and nutrients. The intestinal tract and colon must also be clean.

2.   Optimal health starts with a healthy colon

We are an alchemical factory. Whatever we take into our bodies is converted into the energy required to run our systems. If the food we eat cannot be efficiently processed and eliminated, residue from the alchemical conversion builds up. This residue is toxic if it remains in the body too long. It can be compared to the cold ashes, a dirty house or cluttered hiking trail mentioned in #1.

Detoxing or releasing toxins from the body is a natural biological function. Under optimal conditions, the body needs no assistance in eliminating these toxins. However, today most of us live in a heavily polluted environment. In most areas of the world, the quality of air, water, soil and food has been seriously compromised. Few places on the planet are still pristine and untouched. Heavy metals, parasites and unhealthy bacteria are some of the side effects of living in an impure environment. Fortunately, we have available a number of detoxification programs and products developed by wellness and health conscious individuals that address this challenge.

3.   Any type of blockage in the body systems leads to dis-ease

As conscious beings, we are a combination of physical, mental, emotional and psychological elements. If one or more of these four elements becomes blocked, the body goes into fight or flight (survival) mode. Most people are unaware that the body creates tumors, for example, to store the toxins in an area of the body where they can avoid clogging the body's canals or delivery systems. However, when the tumors grow large enough to interfere with these transportation and communication canals, they start to block the body's normal function.

Anger, fear and other unwanted thoughts, feelings and emotions are also toxic and can cause the same type of blockage as toxic substances or food containing toxins.

4.   Quality food supplements are developed from whole foods

The only supplements that can support the body by cleansing, building and nourishing its cells are derived from whole foods. Any supplement that does not include all the nutrients of the food from which it is extracted cannot possibly support the body systems. Humans can utilize only animal and plant nutrients.

Likewise, supplements that are derived from isolates, inorganic minerals or any other inorganic substance are unable to complement the human diet.

In the next two chapters we will explain in greater detail the difference between disease care and health care.

Chapter 2

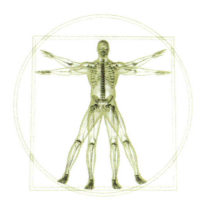

Conventional Medicine – Disease Care

*There are no wonder drugs other than those whose side effects
make you wonder why your doctor prescribed them.*

Challenging medical progress

We all know about the amazing abilities of conventional medicine. We know the lives that have been saved and the suffering that has been alleviated. God help us if we were to live without everything the medical profession provides for us.

My intention in this book is not to challenge the benefits and virtues of conventional medicine, nor to repudiate the thousands of hard-working, devoted and sincere medical doctors and their aides. Our society is deeply indebted to the scientific miracles and highly perfected techniques that succeed in saving many lives, relieving severe distress, addressing extremely complicated crisis and emergency situations and eliminating stressful challenges that would be fatal to many people.

For the moment, however, with great appreciation, let us remove this great profession from its throne and take a look at what it has not succeeded in accomplishing—and at the forces that are holding it back.

In order to properly manage the world of disease, medicine has developed a large number of specialties. Although the sum total of these branches of medicine is significant, it hardly covers the entire spectrum. Medicine is and must remain a profession of disease care.

The study of disease is a full-time and totally absorbing science. No doctor can master all that needs to be known about the manifestations, complications and treatment of disease. Nor can this profession master all that must be known about the world beyond disease—*the world of health.*

Health care is an immense world unto itself. It is not, should not and cannot be within the reach of disease-oriented, disease-trained, and disease-thinking scientists. It is, in fact, unrelated to disease protocols in both practice and research. Health care is an integral part of each of us and because it is, it has to be mastered. It is a world that we must bring close to us in our daily living, thinking, and feeling. It is a challenge to go beyond disease and crisis-care—orthodox or conventional medicine— to *methods and systems of health care.*

There are several reasons for this challenge:
Steady increase of disease.
1. The hazards of drugs.
2. Needless surgery and its hazards.
3. The incompleteness and errors of diagnosis.
4. The ineffectiveness of drug therapies.

Reasons why these challenges still exist:
1. Absence of a solid philosophical basis of medicine.
2. Incomplete insights regarding disease in medical text books.
3. Slow progress.

Conventional medicine has created a paradigm that influences the scientific process by dictating what is studied and researched and also, how the results of the research are interpreted. However, it does not progress toward truths. Rather, it clings to old theories.

Included in this paradigm is the "passing off" of disease care as health care. A deliberate agenda designed by special interest groups promotes this lie and conditions us to buy into it.

Judging from the number of individuals who subscribe wholly to the disease care model of treatment for almost any condition, versus those who have accepted the challenge to start taking responsibility for their health by thinking outside the box (beyond mainstream marketing campaigns), allopathic medicine and its science have been highly successful in winning the popular vote.

Since allopathic prescription medicine is designed and targeted to treat only symptoms, it has no tools for promoting the healing of degenerative or chronic conditions. As a matter of fact, allopathic medicine seldom, if ever, addresses the causes of these conditions. They are generally left untouched and unknown.

You cannot develop a drug unless you have a disease. You cannot have a disease unless you have presenting symptoms.

If a person were to become well—if they were to recover from their chronic conditions—the number of individuals needing prescriptive drugs, hospital stays and surgery would sharply decline. The drug industry's prosperity well would dry up.

Disease is a foreign word to wellness oriented practitioners; it simply does not exist. How could that be?

If we do not categorize symptoms and attach labels to them that can be used as general diagnosis for others who appear to have the same symptoms, we have no basis for giving any particular set of symptoms a name and calling it a "disease." A label does not exist unless we create it.

Why are labels or names and categories important for the medical doctor? Consider: how else would they be able to prescribe a medication according to the PDF or prescription catalog unless they have a set of symptoms that match a particular drug? The recipe must match the symptoms. Thus, the creation of disease is mainly for the purpose of cataloguing data and organizing it in a system that can efficiently serve as the basis for prescribing antidotes or remedies. People often compare a doctor's office to a dispensary or mill: Every 10, 20 or 30 minutes a patient comes in, another patient leaves, each pay at the front desk, and schedule their next appointment.

By creating this paradigm or formula type of treatment, I think we can see how it has influenced the scientific process by dictating what is studied and researched—and also, how the results of the research are interpreted. Instead of progressing toward truths by researching outside the paradigm, it cannot deliver new information or new approaches to treatment. Progress never occurs. It is not intended to.

HOW SCIENTIFIC IS MEDICINE?
How scientific can a profession be when the overall practice is based on principles, diagnostic procedures and therapies that:

- Originated in the age of scientific ignorance, before the nature, structure and functions of cells and biochemistry were known; yet continues even today to promote the same ignorance?

- Disregard the broad range of results of their own medical research and do not incorporate into their philosophy and practices the findings regarding disease and related therapies that are accessible in their libraries and research storehouses?

- Are based solely on partial understandings and even more partial application of the physiology and biochemistry of the human body, mind, and emotions?

- Make little or no attempt to explore and comprehend causal factors of the diseases to be treated?

- Do not treat the causal factors of disease and disregard their nature and importance?

- Treat only those aspects of the disease problems or disabled functions that manifest as symptoms?

- Consider and treat diseases as results of single causes in their most simplified form (e.g., a fracture caused by an accident) and completely ignore the reality of human beings living in a civilization that exposes them to a great number of hazards, pollutants, abnormal lifestyle, stresses, etc.?

- Disregard body pollution and toxicity (including side effects of the drugs they use) as a major cause of most chronic diseases?

- Are based on poisoning the body through the use of drugs, with the deliberate intention of activating resistance to such poisons with hopes that the same body resistance will fight off the diseases?

- Consider everything in the human body as material and chemical, and in so doing, disregard the patterns and principles of life inherent to the nature of human beings?

- Do not hesitate to treat diseases with the same agents that cause these diseases, such as chemotherapy and radiation for the treatment of cancer? Prescribe treatments that are basically limited to drugs, radiation, and surgery?

- Disregard the laws of nature by which all men must live by, breathe and sustain themselves?

- Have no therapy that is capable of curing (completely and totally restoring to normal) any single disease, yet place doctors on a pedestal, touting themselves as the sole authority for all healing?

- Condemn everyone outside the profession of allopathic medicine as ignorant; calling them "quacks" even when centuries of proof support these individuals' knowledge, experience and possession of valuable curative remedies?

- Never look at, diagnose, or provide support for the under-functioning of the liver, which is the sole organ responsible for all healing of the body and normalizing of its functions? (They cannot, because if they understood problems in the liver they would never be able to prescribe drugs as therapies, since every drug damages the liver.)

- Ignore the blatant fact that the benefits of their treatments are merely "band-aids" because they never address the causal factors?

- Corroborate with drug company interests, for developing and maintaining public school health education, academic and vocational school public health and health science training, and medical school curricula– all of which advocate principles and teachings almost identical to those of 80 to 100 years ago?

- Present to the public, images of doctors as healers and scientists capable of restoring heath, but fail to provide patients with the substances (food, herbal, cellular or other concentrates or extracts) – which cells and tissues are unable to regenerate and achieve well-being?

- Persist in their beliefs that there are thousands of incurable diseases—even though almost every disease has already been cured, sometimes centuries ago, by some other therapist using different methods, in another part of the world?

- Have nothing to offer that can cure even one single disease (even though they may perform miracles of emergency care, save lives, restore comfort, and eliminate conditions in the body that are a serious threat to well-being and life itself)?

• Claim that bacteria and viruses are causes of diseases? When researchers (even Pasteur himself declared on his death bed) and research experiments have shown that infectious agents are wise and needy scavengers of body poisons and disease–and they only manifest when the other healing agents of the body fail to control and eliminate the toxins, wastes and debris upon which these bacteria and viruses feed?

Every science-oriented profession, except medicine, has radically changed its basic philosophy to accommodate the vast, ever-increasing influx of knowledge resulting from advanced research and extraordinary breakthrough discoveries. The standard approach to patient care has remained basically the same for the past hundred years.

The medical profession is the most unorthodox of all professions.

The only "orthodox" healing professional is one who considers the full nature and cause of diseases and then treats the total person in harmony with his needs; acting within the scope of the laws of nature and doing NO HARM to any patient.

The scientific approach to health care is holistic, natural, and personal. It addresses the total person. Truth is inescapable and will eventually prevail.

Doctors can dress wounds, but it is nature and the life within us that heals them.

Medical diagnosis

As stated previously, diagnosis in medicine means categorizing or labeling any condition a person may experience. This is where it draws the line. In medical diagnosis, there is no acknowledgment or recognition of the potential value of investigating or evaluating the causes of various diseases, or the processes that took place in the body that created the changes from health to disease. If these processes and causes are not known or treated, how is it possible to cure disease?

The body-mind-emotional triad that is the basic component of every human being is almost infinite in its scope. There is no one profession, body of scientists or group of geniuses that could possibly master the understanding of the total human being or of all the diseases that make him ill.

Post mortem examinations reveal that 50% of diagnoses in all hospitals in America are incorrect or incomplete, which means a person has one chance out of two that their disease is even diagnosed correctly, let alone understood and treated correctly and effectively.

Five minute visits are about as effective for finding the causes of a disease and figuring out a regime of curing, as bringing your car in for an engine overhaul and expecting it to be done in a matter of minutes.

Diseased individuals fill hospital beds and waiting room clinics, while the amazing discoveries resulting from cutting-edge research regarding the nature, processes and causes of disease, fill libraries and the internet.

There are no incurable diseases. There are only incurable people... thousands of them. Among these individuals are those who have passed the point of curability. Others simply don't want to get better; they're ready to leave. Examples of loss of will to live are people who lose a loved one and shortly after become ill and die. Other examples are those who are declared terminal and are brought to a practitioner who uses a different healing modality or technique and these people become miraculously well. The patients with no desire to live will revert to their former condition. Those who are excited and grateful for life extension will live joyously until they really are ready to leave.

Still others don't have the means or the understanding required to properly follow a therapy and benefit completely from its merits. It's too much for them to deal with; for these people it's better to just die and get it over with.

Why do such conditions and ineffectiveness still exist?

As we stated previously, doctors are trained to search for a specific disease, condition or symptom, neatly categorized by the industry, and then from their therapy textbook, find the corresponding "recipe." Since this is the accepted procedure, it is not surprising that it has also been adapted by naturopaths, chiropractors, acupuncturists, herbalists and homeopaths.

In established medicine, the conventional philosophy of disease still claims that every disease is an evil that must be destroyed with drugs, surgery and radiation. They are conditioned to believe that "they" and only "they" have a monopoly on scientific and therapeutic truths.

According to the medical profession there is no other truth and no other healing profession. They have a scientific dictatorship—a monopoly on healing. No other alternative approaches or methods can be allowed.

The present organized controlled system of professional practice was created in the era just before the turn of the 20th century.

Businesses and men of wealth financed the medical schools and set up the therapeutic methods, systems and prototypes. From a practical perspective, medical schools and curricula were organized to teach doctors to quickly and efficiently control and alleviate the symptoms and distresses of workers on assembly lines so their illnesses would not disrupt factory routines and systems as well as business profits. The goal was to keep people functional and working at their jobs without interruption.

In spite of a hundred years of carefully documented knowledge (that is the result of ongoing research conducted by innovative scientists), the basic thinking, parameters and methods of teaching and practicing medicine have not changed beyond the treatment of symptoms, crisis conditions and immediate relief type care.

Doctors are told they are the experts. They "know it all." No scientific knowledge of disease exists outside the medical profession. No person except a doctor has the ability to understand the human body or the material found in scientific textbooks. To this day, this mind conditioning has worked. Standard medicine is a closed loop. Such skewed belief systems have been a great impediment to progress in the medical profession.

Medical Politics

Enforceable laws throughout North America make it illegal for a physician to use any kind of therapy on cancer patients other than drugs, chemotherapy, surgery and radiation. These laws make it a crime to treat patients with new discoveries and treatments. Future therapies will never be acceptable, consequently blocking the possibility of progress in the treatment of cancer.

The parameter of medicine is: toe the line—be orthodox—or be out.

Every medical doctor who has tried to create change, repudiate the ignorance of the past and update science to the new awareness of cell biochemistry and life forces has been persecuted.

Established medicine is the only profession that has failed to evolve in its basic philosophy and principles, which for the most part date back thousands of years. Medical prescriptions are still cookbook recipes for the relief of symptoms. They do not cure and they do not address the cause for the disease.

This stubbornness and stagnation contribute to the dishonor of medical doctors. But are doctors really to blame? Is the deceit intentional? I think not. I believe the vast majority of doctors have a genuine desire to help their patients get better and are hamstrung by the very politics that control their industry and profession.

If there is a culprit, one could point to the drug industry. From a socio-economic and geopolitical standpoint, the name of the game is to create a problem and then develop a profitable business to solve it.

The war machine is a typical example. Start an incursion somewhere and then go in as the peacemaker and sell weapons and industrial tools for building a better society.[2] The drug industry, now integrally linked to the hospital and insurance industries, has

---

2 *Confessions of an Economic Hit Man,* by John Perkins. Plume Press, 2005.

a vested interest in keeping people sick. A person who becomes well, i.e., who no longer needs to buy drugs that can only be prescribed by a medical doctor through a visit to the doctor's office, represents lost profits and a future empty hospital/nursing home bed. Insurance companies lose their edge on selling premiums. Wellness is a liability because it is no longer profitable. Peace is a liability because weapons and "good will intervention" are no longer profitable.[3]

One could even go so far as to say that according to those who hold the purse strings of medicine are the puppet masters of the practitioners—"It is against the law to cure any patient of any disease because this would destroy a huge part of the economy of this great country." They cannot allow that to happen.

Medical schools are geared to select and admit only those students who are achievement oriented and have accumulated top grades, often at the cost of neglecting interpersonal relationships. Doctors are not supposed to empathize and "reach out" to patients in their sufferings. The medical school curriculum dehumanizes even those who come with deeply held ideals and aspirations to serve and assist others.

The history of conventional allopathic medicine

Our current "medical model" or conventional allopathic approach to health stems from one man's view.

This person was Louis Pasteur (1885) who created the "germ theory," the idea that germs are floating around in the air and will attack us if we do not protect ourselves with pharmaceutical substances. Pasteur believed that dangerous germs were the cause of all human disease.

Antoine Beauchamp (1883), an astute research biologist, rejected Pasteur's theory and presented an opposing view. Beauchamp claimed that the "biological terrain" of the afflicted person and not the germ itself is the cause of disease. According to Beauchamp: "The primary cause of disease is always within us."

Beauchamp believed that germs and parasites will only survive in unfavorable conditions. Therefore, mere exposure to germs is not enough to cause illness.

Of the two men's theories, Louis Pasteur's was more popular and more easily accepted. If we could blame disease on germs and not on ourselves, we would no longer have to take responsibility for our own health. This seemed like such an easy solution. Also, it would improve the country's economy, providing thousands with new careers in the manufacturing, marketing, production and promotion of pharmaceuticals.

---

3 http://www.thrivemovement.com/drug-rx-money-making-killing

It has been reported that on his death bed, Pasteur capitulated and agreed that, in fact, Beauchamp's theory was correct, i.e., that all disease begins with the condition of the body. By that time it was too late.

According to Beauchamp, under certain conditions, cells or bacteria of one type can change into cells or bacteria of another. An example of this in human cells might be the morphing of skin cells to connective tissue cells, a typhoid bacillus into a staphylococcus bacteria, or blood cells to bone tissue.

Many in the alternative healing world and even a few on the fringes of conventional mainstream science feel that pleomorphism[4] of microorganisms is widespread, and this is the mechanism that allows nature to perform various tasks of toxic cleanup and tissue removal in the human body. In effect, this theory states that bacteria simply change to whatever form is most readily needed in the body, based on cues from the body itself.

In the many parallel theories of biological terrain assessment and adjustment, the underlying assumption is that "infection" by microorganisms really indicates nothing more than imbalances in the inner biochemical terrain of the body. Thus, if the inner terrain of the body is allowed to normalize, then the "infectious organisms" will cease their inflammatory activity, since their presence is no longer needed.

Bacteria and other microorganisms are not seen as dangerous, invasive pathogens but rather, they are simply responding to cues from the body that cleanup is needed. In other words, they are seen as performing simple but necessary cleanup functions in response to cues from the local body tissues.

Thus, it would make sense that one would treat an infectious illness by simply adjusting the inner terrain of the body to allow it to become more conducive to healthful conditions. This adjustment eliminates the need for the presence of the "infectious" organisms.

Conversely, any attempt to treat an infectious illness with antibiotics (or hydrogen peroxide, ozone or colloidal silver, all of which are favorite therapies in the alternative healing world) would be seen in most cases as short-sighted. The practitioner would be attempting to treat a symptom of imbalance, rather than address the actual imbalance.

Further, this theory would suggest that most, if not all, antibiotics and other aggressive antimicrobial agents would actually lead to even greater imbalance and disruption of natural body functions. The end result would be further degeneration.

---

4 The occurrence of more than one different form in the life cycle of a plant or animal
http://www.thefreedictionary.com/pleomorphism

Chapter 3

The Wellness Model – Health Care

Only nature can cure…
No remedy is going to work for you if you do nothing to help yourself.

As we stated previously, healthy living and enjoyment of life is a matter of achieving and maintaining balance:

- Emotional
- Physical and structural
- Work and play
- Habits
- Mindsets

Healthy balance is:

- The integrity, strength and effectiveness of our nerves and nervous system, which control our organs, tissues and glands.
- The proper functioning of all glands and organs.
- The presence of all hormones in proportions required for controlling and balancing all body biochemicals.
- The presence of all enzymes required for every function of living in balance.
- The presence of acid and alkaline substances in our body tissues and cells that can create the proper environment for the perfect functioning and activities of all enzymes.

The proper positioning and inter-relationship of bones and muscles, creating balanced structural and body movements.

Humans are not machines

Contrary to the allopathic or conventional medical model, we humans are so much more than machines with parts that can be "fixed" or "replaced."

The vital force of our body systems depends on *six dynamic processes* working together synergistically and harmoniously.

Those processes are:

Chemical	Electric
Nutrient-Electronic	Magnetic
Oxidative	Atomic

1. Chemical

Digestion of food is a chemical process that provides the body systems with all the basic nutrients needed for building, repairing and regenerating cells. Our teeth chew and crumble food that is then macerated or liquefied into tiny nutrient molecules by digestive enzymes secreted by our glands.

The different molecular substances in foods inter-react and release chemical energy. As this chemical process is repeated, it continues to release even more energy.

One of the final steps of food breakdown occurs in the intestines as molecules are split off from the original food morsels. The cells prepare the sugar and transform it into molecular nutrients which they will use as fuel or life force energy.

2. Nutrient-Electronic Energy

In the structures of all nutrient molecules and atoms are tiny satellite type fragments called electrons. In miniature, they are like the moon that circles the earth. Electrons are coupled to the atoms by the same type of magnetic force that holds planets in their respective positions.

When electrons separate from their mother atom, (a process called "fission") they release nutrient-electronic energy that becomes available as life force energy.

In our daily diets we take in the same nutrient elements that we eliminate in our body wastes. This is not a useless or excessive quirk of nature. Our bodies replenish themselves daily with these nutrient rich foods in order to acquire the electrons or nutrient-electronic energy from the minerals found in these foods.

3. Oxidation Energy

The oxidation process is like oxygen acting on wood burning in a fireplace, although without a flame. Heat is essential to cell life and contributes to the production of life force energy. When the sugars, oils, fats and proteins of our food combine with oxygen, they become *fuel foods* and create calories.

4.   Electrical Energy

Electricity is one of our main sources of life and energy. Body cells are actually batteries. It takes the presence of an acid–acting on two different chemical substances to create an electrical charge. The nuclei of all cells are like the negative poles, and the colloidal and liquid substances (protoplasm or living matter) are like the positive poles. In our body cells, the acid is hydrochloric acid, normally secreted by the stomach. When charged, our cells become trillions of microscopic life and energy generating batteries.

Hydrochloric acid is a normal stomach secretion. It is not usually considered by the medical industry to be important in the treatment of diseases. Yet, a deficiency of hydrochloric acid may cause every cell to go into energy decline. Our bodies will experience fatigue or exhaustion. The cells degenerate, losing their ability to use proteins and minerals and function normally.

About 10% of children are born with an inability to secrete sufficient amounts of hydrochloric acid. Over ninety percent of all people with cancer are deficient in hydrochloric acid.

5.   Magnetic Energy

The world is a magnet. All minerals—even oxygen—are magnets. Attraction between nutrient molecules and the cell walls bring nutrients to the cells. These nutrients cannot enter the cells, nor can the cells use them unless their magnetic properties are active. Thus, the magnetic forces of the body become an expression of their life and energy.

Magnetism also plays a role in the elimination of cell waste and debris, thus helping to keep the cells healthy. By magnetic attraction, all used up elements inside the cells are drawn to the cell membranes where the refuse is eliminated. Magnetic energies and vibrations enhance both immunity and healing.

6.   Atomic Energy

Atomic research has demonstrated that matter doesn't exist, i.e., that matter is condensed energy. With knowledge such as this, now known for generations, why are doctors still using chemicals and drugs as therapies? Why are they not using energies, life forces and therapeutic frequencies?

The very nature of the cells themselves sends us this message.

NOTE: Any depletion of these life forces can be a serious hazard to health and a contributing cause to severe chronic degenerative diseases, including cancer, AIDs, etc.

Only nature can cure

Medicine and surgery can remove obstructions, but neither can cure. *Only nature can cure.* Surgery removes the bullet, but nature heals the wound.

Conventional medicine covers up the symptoms of a serious disease. This leads to more degeneration and disease, and as stated previously, recurring doctors' visits, more tests, hospital stays, etc. A person becomes a permanent patient. The *causes* of the disease, which are the symptoms or signs, e.g., toxins, metabolic and retained wastes and unhealthy foods, are covered up by pain medication. The toxins and other causes remain untreated.

If suppressed and allowed to accumulate, all abnormal substances (e.g., toxins and unhealthy foods) slowly destroy the body. Systemic toxicity develops into any number of challenging diseases, such as arthritis, cancer, heart disease and many other degenerative conditions. These are the conditions that afflict almost half the population in America.

We can't put the blame on our physicians for destroying us. We did it to ourselves, usually with our favorite "poison": cigarettes, ice cream, sugar, alcohol, etc. A negative mindset, such as anger, fear, worry, resentment, stress or self-neglect, can also have the same effect.

The moment a person suppresses their authentic or real nature, whether to please someone or refrain from displeasing them, they compromise their body-mind emotional integrity. If this behavior becomes habitual, the body systems start to deteriorate. Disease is the inevitable outcome.

There are NO incurable diseases

Anyone can be well. You have to take control of your destiny and your physical, mental and emotional state of being. However, if out of ignorance or neglect you allow a condition with presenting symptoms to progress to an incurable state, you WILL become a candidate for the inevitable consequences.

Most of you know by now, either from personal experience or witnessing the lifestyles and habits of others, that excessive behavior, negligence or failure to take care of your body's needs, and habitual self-abuse (chemical, substance and food addictions, for example; or chronic conditions of anger, resentment, guilt, jealousy, etc.) will have an adverse effect on your health, your daily life, your relationships and your career or business.

In order to enjoy optimum wellness and experience physical, mental and emotional fitness, you must first accept responsibility for your own healing and provide your body with everything that is required to restore well-being. You must accept and appreciate that you need help, such as guidance, support and the right remedies. Denial or avoidance of presenting symptoms is another form of negligence or abuse, even if it may not seem as overt.

You also need a clear understanding of the full nature of your disease: what you have to cure is YOU. **You are not a label for a diagnosed illness or condition.** Remember: Conventional medical labels are nothing more than the name of a specific disease pattern that is derived from statistics in a data base.

You are not a statistic. You are a unique human being.

Believe in your wellness program

Regardless of the treatment or therapy you have chosen for addressing your challenge, it is important that you are totally committed to it—that you believe in it 100%.

It is important to understand and accept that curing is NOT what your doctor is doing for you by removing or destroying organs as if they were only spare parts of little value, or by prescribing drugs. Drugs may have the capacity to make you feel better… not BE better.

No doctor or drug has ever cured a single person of any type of disease. No remedy or treatment can guarantee magic elimination of disease and complete restoration of health. **No medicine has magical powers.** There are no healing panaceas or wonder drugs other than those whose side effects make you wonder why your doctor prescribed them in the first place.

No remedy is going to work for you if you do nothing to help yourself. Like everything in nature, if your condition is neglected for too long, you may have missed your chance for restoration. Cures don't work if you have neglected your body's needs beyond the point of no return.

Curing is not just bandaging, relieving or controlling symptoms.

Curing is:

1. The restoration of the wholeness and perfection of YOU…
    » Your body and mind.
    » Your emotions and life forces.
    » Your purpose of living.
    » Your ability to live intensely.
    » Your peace of mind and joy of living.
    » The neutralizing and elimination of all toxins
2. The replenishing of all nutrients and body needs.
3. Utilization of those therapies that really cure, whether natural, alternative or holistic.

The 3 C's of curing:
- CARING
- CLEANING
- CHANGING

Caring

Caring is more than merely taking the pills the doctor prescribed and/or all those vitamins and supplements you believe to be good for you.

It is more than "watching your diet" according to what your mother served at home or what TV has taught you. It is more than jogging or exercising and working out.

"Caring meals" are not breakfasts of coffee, toast, corn flakes, milk and sugar; lunches consisting of a sandwich and a bowl of canned soup; and a dinner of very well cooked meat, mashed potatoes, canned or frozen vegetables… or if in a hurry, a TV dinner, pizza or Big Mac.

Caring for yourself also means making time to "chill out" and relax. It is so important to enjoy yourself and also make the effort to find out exactly what your whole person needs. Do you need to take a walk and get away from the computer? Get some sunshine? Spend time with a good friend?

It is often said that some people pay more attention to their lawns, house interiors or vehicles and take better care of them than they take care of themselves. You keep your prize possessions in excellent condition. You spend time and energy learning how to give them the best care. If you were to have a luxury car you would most assuredly give it special care. You would regularly change the oil and clean the air and oil filters. You wouldn't consider filling your tank with cut-rate gas. You would keep the right amount of air in the tires and service it on a regular basis.

Why not give the same attention to yourself?

If you were to own an expensive racehorse, would you be keeping him up half the night partying? Would you be feeding him junk food and forcing him to smoke cigarettes? I don't think so.

Why, then, do we give so much care and attention to those things that, although they may have value, can never compare to the value of our minds, our bodies, our feelings and our physical abilities? Our body, mind, spirit and emotions are our sacred temple with all the marvels and creations of God's miracle within. It is up to us to be good caretakers and stewards of that temple.

Cleaning

Body toxicity is a major part of all serious illness. Did you know that since 1945, no civilized individual has lived a single minute of their lives free of chemicals, drugs, pollutants and poisons?

In 1945 drug companies took over the marketplace—and our lives. In preparation for ongoing warfare, U.S. warehouses were filled with tens of thousands of tons of chemicals and drugs. With no way to dispose of them, the companies that manufactured these lethal substances dumped them into our country's waterways, air, soil—and our human bodies.

We now live in a world infiltrated with tens of thousands of toxic and hazardous chemicals and pollutants.

Every drug that is prescribed for you by a doctor is a hazard to your health because it is a poison.

There is no such thing as a humanly processed tablet, pill or capsule that does not have some harmful effect on our body.

Every unnatural and processed substance, every chemical, everything that man touches or changes, is toxic.

One out of three people who show up in hospital emergency rooms are there because of damaging side effects from prescription drugs. Let's repeat this another way: *One out of three individuals on prescription drugs (prescribed by a medical doctor) experiences adverse side effects--and requires emergency care.*

Changing

In the early part of the last century, J. H. Tilden, a medical physician, abandoned the use of drugs after 18 years of practice. He claimed that not only did drugs fail to cure disease; they also promoted or contributed to it! Dr. Tilden started treating his patients based on his Theory of Toxemia. Later he published a book, *Toxemia Explained.*

Since ancient times, the theory of body toxicity and detoxification has been the basis of certain healing practices. The word "toxemia" means poisons *(tox)* in the blood *(emia)*. Dr. Tilden's use of the toxemia also referred to poisons saturating body fluids and blood as well as tissues and cells throughout the body.

Dr. Tilden's discussion of toxemia is simple and concise. He clearly explains how we develop many diseases, and offers methods for regaining health and preventing further illness.

According to Dr. Tilden, toxemia is the result of living in an unhealthy environment—constant exposure to toxins, pollutants and hazardous chemicals. Negative thoughts, values, attitudes, habits and lifestyles also contribute to toxicity. Our bodies become overwhelmed by the huge influx of abnormal chemicals, drugs and pollutants. These poisons accumulate and stagnate in our blood and tissue fluids. Our cells bathe in these fluids like fish in an ocean.

For comparison, consider a small pond where various plants, fish, frogs and crickets thrive. Under ideal conditions, fresh water is always circulating in the pond. Outflow transports wastes and pollutants produced by animals and plants, and inflow delivers clean water.

If the pond's inflow and outflow of water become sluggish or blocked, the water stagnates. Waste collects. Gradually vibrant health of the pond declines. The lilies become soggy and covered with slime; the fish swim listlessly, if at all, and the frogs no longer croak. The shore and floor of the pond become covered with a brown muck and the once crystal-clear water becomes dark and smells foul. Possibly you've seen—and smelled—a stagnant pond.

This filthy, dismal condition of a stagnant pond is analogous to the body of the average middle-aged patient. His body produces wastes and cell debris faster than it can dispose of them. Just like the pond, this waste and debris stagnate in his blood and tissue fluids.

When a person's throat is sore, it isn't because it has been attacked by vicious germs. Microbes or disease-causing bacteria generally aren't aggressive invaders; they fall into holes in our tissues that were dug by toxins that have stagnated in our body.

According to Tilden's theory, a sore throat is caused by the poisoning of throat cells and tissues that are unable to resist penetration by microbes. If we have a sore throat, unless we flush our mouths with an odor-killing solution, our breath has a stench as offensive as the foul odor of a stagnant pond.

Arthritis is not due to the "wear-and-tear" of our joints but to toxic wastes that accumulate in the joint tissues. With toxic buildup, joint tissues cannot cope even with normal joint stress. The joints degenerate because they are unable to repair themselves. Movements then severely irritate the joint tissues. They become inflamed, swollen and painful.

When we pass foul smelling gas, it's not because we ate the wrong type of beans (this may contribute a little), or swallowed too much air (not likely) but because toxic wastes in blood that flows through the tissues of the stomach and intestinal walls have poisoned their cells. In chain reaction, sluggish or blocked cellular activity suppresses the secretion of enzymes necessary for the complete digestion of all foods.

Foods that are not completely digested rot and putrefy, generating gases with foul odors. As these rotting or putrefying substances slowly pass through the intestines, they are absorbed into the bloodstream. This completes the vicious cycle of toxicity by again poisoning the digestive organs. The intestines become a cesspool and sewage system, a source of disease for the rest of the body. The toxin saturated blood travels to every organ, tissue and cell of the body, delivering its poisons wherever it goes.

When wastes accumulate to a high concentration, they "intoxicate" or poison our cells. This toxicity can affect the brain, causing a person to feel sluggish, emotionally depressed and irritable. It can affect the muscles, especially heart muscles, making a person feel weak and lethargic. Toxic skin becomes sallow and wrinkled. Glandular toxicity upsets nerves and emotions, leaving a person tired, unhappy and without a sex drive. Toxicity is an open invitation for infections and disease.

If we truly want to enjoy optimum wellness, these toxic cycles must be eliminated. In order to achieve body balance and efficient function, *toxins must be flushed from the system*. Even the best body cleansing products are useless unless we stop adding toxins to the body, and until we get rid of all pollutants. This is done by a process called *detoxification.*

Mother Nature is a benevolent tyrant

Every cell, organ, fluid and structural part of our body is a masterpiece of perfection. The enjoyment of wellness demands that they be kept in this state. Every component must be maintained at the highest level of structural integrity. Every vital force and energy reserve must be sustained at their peak performance. Every biochemical must be in plentiful supply and in balance.

Throughout our lifetime the integrity and identity of our whole being must be preserved according to our specific individuality. All body needs must be provided for. Reserves of every biochemical nutrient and element that participate in the performance of millions of intricate functions of living must be kept at their maximum, or their supply must be constantly replenished. Failure to do so is certain to bring upon our bodies, minds and emotions the wrath of distress, discomfort, disability, and eventually the onset of disease.

Mother Nature is a benevolent tyrant. She demands to be treated with justice and consideration at all times, and to be appreciated, respected and revered. She handsomely rewards those who honor her and furnish her with all her needs.

Mother Nature heals, repairs and restores in so many miraculous ways. However, she can and will be cruel to those who tend to abuse her. She will not hesitate to manifest abuse in distressful, painful and cruel ways.

Our bodies do not make mistakes. Every process in the body follows the same pattern of perfection. Nature devises and creates mechanisms that are uncanny, ingenious and generous beyond the call of duty. She constantly seeks and finds miraculous ways of compensating, correcting, normalizing and restoring our bodies to their original state of integrity. Although she is our greatest healer, at a certain point she can become so tightly shackled she will lose her healing abilities.

Poisons are Nature's shacklers

The symptoms, upheavals and distresses that manifest as illnesses are not devils. They are not forms of punishment or evil "hexes." Rather, they are a part of Nature's ingenious, highly beneficent warning system. They are "red lights" that alert us when an organ or body function is seriously threatened by potential damage or disease.

Fatigues, weaknesses, aches, pains, cramps, fevers, diarrheas, tumors, dizzy spells and other symptoms are not diseases. They are always the best and most effective way— sometimes the only available way—to warn our bodies that they need to defend, protect and repair themselves. They are signals for getting rid of causes, mobilizing healing processes, eliminating threats and detoxifying and neutralizing toxins and poisons; at least until other means can be brought into play to support our bodies in their effort to return their systems to a state of balance.

Healing is an ongoing event

Your body is constantly in a state of healing. It simply *cannot stop* healing. If you need more proof of this, test the healing process on your own skin with a slight cut or a small drop of a mild acid. Or, place your hand lightly over a hot stove burner. Protect the damaged skin from further irritation or cover it to prevent it from becoming infected. Then notice that you cannot stop your wound from healing. You can continue to damage a wound faster than it can heal by scratching and irritating it, then allowing it to become infected. Even the infection will not stop the healing process.

Healing has a multitude of symptoms or indicators. Rarely does one need to keep repeating blood tests and X-rays or getting monthly follow-up examinations and other tests. Listen to the quiet songs of increasing wellness from the body itself. Believe in them. Know they are telling you constantly that you are feeling better and happier than before.

You feel a release from anxieties, with less tension throughout your body. You are starting to relax a little better. Your head feels lighter. Your sleeping has improved. You function better. Your mind works better. Your body is more limber. You are more energetic and less irritable.

You start to feel more like yourself, with less aches and decreased pain, or maybe none at all. Any growths that may have started, have decreased in size; sores or eruptions are disappearing.

You don't need a doctor to tell you that you're improving, nor do you need to collect a pile of laboratory tests and proofs for confirmation.

As long as you are experiencing these positive, healing signs of release, relaxation, flow and "lightness of being" with improved function, there's no way that any disease can possibly maintain its foothold and independently survive. It is not possible to have health and disease at the same time, nor is it possible to experience healing and worsening simultaneously. You cannot do everything that your body needs in order to heal, and not experience this healing!

This rule of Mother Nature is true even when you experience periods of feeling worse, as if a relapse is occurring and your illness is starting over again or getting worse. *While following a regime that corresponds to your body's healing needs, your body cannot get worse.* However, your body can attack storage areas in your tissues where it has deposited wastes and debris, toxins and body pollutants. It will release this toxic waste into your bloodstream in order to get rid of it permanently.

Dumping toxins back into your body causes you to feel sick or actually become sick, just as if you were to eat poisoned food, take a strong drug or alcoholic drink. It doesn't matter how you poison yourself; *you will feel poisoned.* The feeling will be the same, but inside something altogether different is occurring. Often this feeling is referred to as a "healing crisis."

If you are poisoning your system by deliberately ingesting or imbibing poison, you are creating a toxic body. On the other hand, if you are detoxifying your body by following a healing regime, you will be removing toxins that are already in the body systems. The process of eliminating those toxins as they flow into the bloodstream will feel exactly the same, since in both instances, your body is dealing with toxins. If you are healing and eliminating toxins, your condition is not worse. You are simply experiencing a symptom of "the worst (toxins) coming out."

Each time you experience a dumping of toxins, there will be less toxins left to dump. Each healing crises will be less severe than the previous one and the intervals between will become longer. You will know what they are and what to do about them, so you will not be anxious when they occur. As you flush out the toxic wastes you will quickly and efficiently control and eliminate the severity.

During periods of healing from a serious or long illness, it is not uncommon to experience the recurrence of some other illness or problem similar to and reminiscent of a health problem from an earlier time in your life.

If adequate measures were not taken at that time to completely eliminate the causes of that previous illness or if drugs suppressed the factors that caused it, thus blocking the body's ability to release them (drugs tend to suppress causal factors), and your body has successfully healed your present illness, it will attack those buried causal factors. Nature is such a powerful healer, it will resurrect the former problem and continue to repair and restore each of the body systems until everything returns to normal.

Re-experiencing former illnesses does not mean you are "getting them again." Rather, it means you are "getting at them" to get rid of them, once and for all! Often people refer to this experience as "peeling the onion." Like an onion that grows in many layers that can be peeled down to the core, you are peeling off all the inner layers of suppressed causal factors and healing each of them, one at a time, until finally you reach, and heal the core issue.

Healing takes time

Healing always proceeds at the same speed as growing. Your body heals as fast as it took to grow from being a teenager into an adult. There is no way to make it heal faster. Getting rid of causal factors and toxins can happen rapidly. You may feel better immediately. However, as the body settles down in its attempt to keep the systems balanced, so does your rate of healing.

Points to remember

- Healing is one of Mother Nature's many miracles.

- Healing requires tuning in to yourself in order to understand how the process works and what is involved.

- Healing requires believing in yourself and in your body.

- Healing requires being true to yourself and being faithful to your body's needs.

- Healing takes patience. When going through the healing process, you need to have faith. You have to learn to believe in your body and realize it is a treasure trove of healing potentials and miracles.

Chapter 4

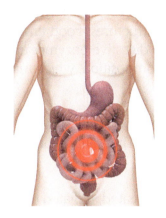

The Cause of Dis-ease

Intestinal Toxicity

The 5 basic sources and types of intestinal pollution are:

1. Failure to digest all food.
2. Excess intake of junk food, dead food, synthetic food, overcooked food and food that has been chemically treated.
3. Ingestion of toxic substances, chemicals and drugs.
4. Prolonged stagnation of fecal waste by constipation.
5. Negative or unwanted mindsets that have a toxic impact on the nervous system; examples are: anger, fear, anxiety, hatred, resentment, and stress.

Our foods contain up to 3,000 chemicals. Almost every food we normally buy at the grocery store has poisons in it: a pesticide, chemical fertilizer, or fancy chemical coloring, flavoring or sweetener. They are all toxic. We are conditioned to believe that foods treated with chemical preservatives will retain their goodness. "Preservative" is merely a pleasant sounding word for "food embalming substance."

Just as an undertaker embalms a corpse, so does a preservative embalm our food. These chemicals destroy the life force and nutritional value of the food. However, their destructive action doesn't stop there. After they are ingested, they proceed to damage our body fluids, blood, oxygen, cells and hormones, until they are eliminated.

To avoid intestinal pollution, we must first understand how the digestive process works.

All living foods consist of cells, and all cells contain hundreds of thousands of enzymes. When these cells start to die, i.e., cease to function, the enzymes break down the cell components and structures. Food enzymes actually digest up to 75% of themselves before the body's digestive enzymes are called into action. This auto-destruct mechanism creates decomposition, which turns to compost which the body excretes.

A miraculous "wisdom" in the body's digestive enzymes prevents them from attacking normal healthy living body cells. They attack only cells that are auto-destructing, dying or dead.

Foods that have been chemically treated, radiated or overcooked cannot decompose because their enzymes have been destroyed.

Body toxicity is a major part of all serious illness for those residing in a polluted environment. As stated earlier, since 1945, the year that drug companies took over the marketplace, none of us living in civilized sectors of the world has experienced a single minute of our lives free of chemicals, drugs, pollutants and poisons.

We live in a toxic world. Our air is constantly inundated with smog, fumes and pollutants. In our homes we breathe in more chemicals from aerosols, building materials, furniture, drapes and carpets. Our clothes, shoes, accessories, work and recreational materials, machines and devices—everything contains chemicals or harmful substances.

Our environment is saturated up to three times the human tolerance level with radiation. The body absorbs these airborne toxins much more readily and rapidly even than the chemicals in our food and water.

In most cities, the beautiful crystal clear water we drink and that is so essential to life is loaded with fluorides. Fluorides are fifteen times more poisonous than arsenic; they are the most powerful destroyer of all enzymes. Some city water contains up to fifty or more additional diabolical poisons, even dioxins, which are known to cause cancer.

Doctors seldom warn us about these poisons. When prescribing drugs for us to take, rarely do they tell us how harmful they are. In fact, they never consider them the cause for most diseases, especially cancer, AIDS, chronic fatigue syndrome, obesity, liver disease, headaches and most of our other aches and pains. It is a proven fact that there is a direct correlation between prescriptive drug use and those who manifest every known chronic degenerative disease. In our current state of pollution—our bodies, foods, water and air are polluted by chemicals and other toxins. Our minds and emotions are polluted by TV, crime, politics and financial challenges. We do little, if anything, to counteract this onslaught.

Toxic minds cause disease

It is possible that the single most insidious destructive agent on the planet is a negative mindset. Almost all of these highly destructive negative emotions, such as anxiety, anger, stress, worry etc., can be directly attributed to one culprit: FEAR. Fear is the single most disintegrating factor in human personality.

Ancient cavemen depicted worry by drawing pictures on their cave walls of a wolf sinking its fangs into a man's throat. The word "worry" comes from an old Anglo-Saxon word meaning "to strangle or choke." The effect of fear on the mind and emotions is similar to the physical experience of having one's windpipe crushed and thus blocking off all oxygen intake. This is one of the reasons why meditation and other ways to connect with the Source or one's higher self are so valuable to health and well-being. These activities and practices purge the mind of toxic or destructive thoughts and feelings.

In our current state of pollution—our bodies, foods, water and air polluted by chemicals and other toxins; and our minds and emotions polluted by TV, crime, politics and financial challenges—we do little, if anything, to counteract this onslaught.

Many of us are conscientious about taking our daily regimen of vitamins and minerals, believing these will maintain or restore our health. However, unless made from complete, whole foods, they are dead chemicals. Almost all of these products are manufactured by a drug company.

With the overload of poison entering our bodies, few of us take any measures to release it. Almost no one goes on a fast or uses detoxifying herbs or enemas to neutralize, purge and eliminate the huge overload of toxic substances that saturate our bodies.

Most of us don't have frequent enough bowel movements to get rid of our ordinary daily body and food wastes along with debris of dying cells and accumulated pollutants.

Thanks to poor detoxification and bowel elimination, these poisons stagnate in our systems. They continue to accumulate until the day comes when their amount surpasses levels of body tolerance. The cells and tissues break down and we get sick.

Chapter 5

Pain: Its Nature & Causes

All pains are triggered by the action of anything abnormal that contacts nerve endings in the areas where pain is experienced. The tips of the nerves are sensitive surfaces. When body wastes, chemicals, drugs, physical blows, any type of damage, pressure, or excessive temperatures contact these sensor areas, they send out SOS signals. These signals go directly to the brain.

Pain is a warning, a type of "red-light" that poisons are present or that nerve endings are being damaged, irritated, or undergoing pressure. The pain signals awaken our body's reflexes and force us to act in ways that will avoid or correct the condition. This is our body's normal and essential mechanism for self-protection. Routine use of pain killers is like living close to a fire house and after dealing with the 24/7 annoyance of the siren for awhile (the pain), you sneak over one dark night and cut its wires. Unfortunately, the next fire may be in your own house (your body) and no one will respond because the siren ("pain alarm") never goes off.

The Relief of Distresses & Pains

Detoxifying enzymes can control the distresses and "horror symptoms" commonly associated with many of the disease conditions.

With the exception of pain caused by pressure on nerves, poison neutralization and elimination can relieve pain better than the pain killing drugs. Intense, prolonged detoxification can also relieve extremely severe pain for which even morphine is incapable of providing relief.

When necessary, the body actually can produce its own pain killers (encephalin and endorphins) that are many times stronger than anything the drug store has to offer. This is how athletes "hit the wall," feeling they can't go on because of the pain. Yet if they push just a little harder, these substances are released and they go into a state of almost painless euphoria. Since the body has manufactured these substances, it also knows how to eradicate them at the proper time.

A drug company cannot obtain a patent for a substance that has always existed in nature; therefore, they must change the molecule into something that has never existed before. This changed molecule is called an "analogue."[5]

Nature threw the drug companies a curve, however. If they change 10% of the molecule, 10% of its function now differs from the natural or original molecule. This is one of the major causes of every drug's adverse side effects.

A second problem relates to the fact that the body's detoxification mechanisms have never encountered this molecule before. Therefore, it has no experience in detoxifying it. This places an additional strain on the body system at the precise time when less stress is a key factor in healing enhancement.

Any regime that effectively eliminates toxins, drugs and body poisons provides pain relief for patients with disease conditions.

If the substances that notify nerve endings of their presence are not extremely irritating or toxic, the signals they send to the brain will not necessarily be associated with pain. Symptoms and re-actions may be felt as discomfort, distress, fatigue, malaise, headache, irritability, up-tightness, anxiety, sleeplessness, a mental dullness, depression, or a hangover-like sensation.

---

5 Something that bears an analogy to something else, http://www.thefreedictionary.com/analogue

Chapter 6

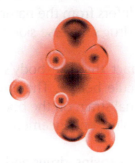

The World of Living Cells

In this chapter we will pay homage to the world of living cells. We will appreciate its wonders, reflect on its myriad of intricate interactions, visualize how a cell component and molecule work intimately together, and allow ourselves to become their students.

Cells have many valuable lessons to teach us. The messages they offer can serve as blueprints and guidelines for healing, and for the selection of wellness therapies. Most of these lessons have yet to be incorporated in a medical doctor's formal training. A brief review of the world of cells could be a good reminder of its forgotten wonders.

Today most healing modalities and various related professions still focus almost solely on the physical body's structures, functions and chemistry. Even in this so-called era of enlightenment, diseases are still considered evils to be suppressed or destroyed by weapons (remedies) specific to each condition. Rather than aiming to heal or "make whole" by restoring cellular abnormality in structure and function to its original stage of integrity, practitioners tend to treat patients and clients according to recipes or formulas. They treat "problems" and not people.

As discussed previously, doctors, casual therapists, health stores and those who sell and use vitamins, minerals and other nutritional products, have "disease recipe books." Too much diagnosis and therapy is based on guesswork rather than knowledge of each individual and the condition of his cells. "Such and such symptoms and problems" are treated by "such and such diet or supplements."

What follows is not to be considered a scientific treatise, nor is it altogether accurate or complete. A library of volumes would be required to make such a presentation. I do not expect this book to change the philosophy and practices that have been deeply ingrained in our current professional system for over centuries. Hopefully, however, this review of the nature of cells may provoke renewed thought about the potential for revising and thus improving current therapeutic approaches.

Cells and human beings are infinitely complex. Their structures consist of thousands of biochemicals. They vary infinitely in the nature of their composition and in the manifestation of the many diseases that afflict them.

The nature and intricacies of the impact of toxicities and deficiencies on cells remains complex and mysterious. Understanding disease on the cellular level is an exciting challenge but it is the path we need to travel if we really want to succeed in eliminating disease.

Where do you find the truth when:

- Doctors claim they cannot discover what's wrong with you—when your body is sending signals of definite distress but the doctors claim you have no illness?

- One doctor says this is the problem, and another says, "No, your illness is something else," and a third doctor claims something altogether different?

- Doctors of one profession claim doctors of other professions are not qualified healers because those doctors' training is different from their own?

- Doctors claim doctors of other professions are wrong and call them quacks?

- The so-called orthodox doctors claim that only drugs have a therapeutic value, when all drugs are poisons and thus the cause of disease; how can poisonous substances restore cells to health?

- Some doctors say vitamins and minerals work miracles and others say they are incapable of curing any disease?

- It is well known that 50% of all diagnoses made by the so-called expert M.D.s are mistakes?

- Differences of professional beliefs foster incompatible attitudes, mutual criticisms, controversies and condemnations?

- Almost every health book we read offers ideas and beliefs different from every other health book?

Almost all of the above problems stem from the following:

1. Most serious, long term, degenerative and so-called incurable diseases are those that have damaged or destroyed cells or the biochemicals by which our cells and bodies function.

2. Over the past centuries little or no accurate, complete or scientific knowledge of the nature, biochemistry or functioning of cells existed.

As a result of these two problems, most genuine understanding of disease was not possible. Consequently, most professional and even so-called scientific opinions were based on conjecture, incomplete knowledge and guesswork. Unless opinions, diagnoses and therapies are based on and confirmed by cell science, opinions of doctors still have the same value as those adhered to during the previous centuries of ignorance.

Professionals and doctors don't like to admit any form of ignorance. They are trained and conditioned to believe and have confidence in their judgments and expertise. Anyone who differs from their beliefs "must" be wrong, misinformed, ignorant or classified as a quack.

Our bodies consist of several hundred different types of cells: nerve, brain, skin, muscle, blood, stomach, liver, pancreas, kidney, lung, heart, etc. Each cell type has its own specific shape and structure, and each cell constituent has its own specific set of functions. All of these biochemicals only function optimally when they are in state of harmony with themselves and other body biochemicals.

Cells are microscopically small in size. Hundreds to thousands of cells can fit comfortably onto the head of a pin. Each is very complex and intricate—a little world unto itself. It is difficult for us to visualize living creations that can be so tiny, yet this is another miracle of Mother Nature.

If broken down even further, one discovers that each cell is comprised of many hundreds of thousands of molecules. All of these molecules are systematically organized into hundreds of minute structures called *organelles*. Each organelle performs a number of chemical functions that are responsible for sustaining human life and creating its miracles.

Cellular research is a massive undertaking. It has required massive teams of scientists merely to describe the amazing aspects of cells. Even though their research would already fill several huge libraries, they are well aware that they have yet to master their secrets, of which it is believed to be well over several million.

Cell Components

Every cell structure and organelle consists of building blocks. The raw materials of these blocks are proteins and minerals.

Proteins with minerals form the skeletal structure of cells as well as the structures of chromosomes and enzymes. These blocks are comprised of approximately 30 amino acids.

All cells require energy for their function and fuel to maintain their temperature. Sugars and oils supply each, respectively.

Sugars in the forms of glycogen granules and cantharides are the source of molecules. When a molecule splits, it releases energy for cell function. All body biochemicals must be utilized in harmony with cellular needs, which require proper balance. Balance and cell protection are the responsibilities of quality oils.

Oils are the raw materials from which the endocrine glands manufacture hormones, whose role it is to keep all of the body's biochemicals, functions, growing patterns and nutrient utilization in balance.

Oils also form a protective coating around cells. Similar to oil that protects your skin from the excessive rays of sunshine and sunburn, cell oils form part of the cell membrane and protect the cells from the harmful effects of body wastes, toxins, drugs, chemicals, and poisons.

Oils come in various formulas of 3-6 fatty acids: neutral lipids, cholesterol, oleic acid, linoleic acid, and arachidonic acid. Each plays a special role.

Lecithin-Phospholipids, together with amino-acids, trace minerals, and oils create the membranes of cells that form the outer sack. Lecithin links the oils to the water soluble elements, thereby reinforcing the protective coating of cells.

Gross Minerals:

- **Potassium** is the main mineral ingredient of cells. It stabilizes acid-alkalinity.

  Potassium also normalizes cell chemistry, stabilizes and slows growth and division of cells, and contributes to the functioning and intensity of cell function.

- **Sodium** affects cells from their outside. When combined with a hydrogen and oxygen molecule linked together, it acts as a stimulant to cells. This stimulant also activates the multiplication of cells. When in excess it enters the cells and brings water with it. This causes the cells to swell. Increased volume of cells also activates cell division.

- **Calcium** creates strength and solidity of cells, especially those that form the brittle skeletal tissues, such as bones and teeth. Calcium is also a carrier of the electric messages that travel through the nerves and create communication between our brains and every other tissue of the body.

- **Phosphorus** helps solubilize calcium and other minerals so they will be in a form that can be readily used by cells.

Trace Minerals:

When combined with amino acids, trace minerals create the mitochondria bodies of cells and the enzymes whereby they function within the cells.

Trace minerals together with amino acids also form the chromosomes which then fabricate the enzymes whereby the cells function and grow. Each trace mineral works singly or in groups for each specific organ, and in this manner contributes to their specific functions.

- **Iron** comprises red blood cells and carries oxygen.
- **Cobalt** is essential to the formation of red blood cells.
- **Iodine** is an essential part of thyroid hormones.
- **Magnesium** enhances the action of calcium and helps slow down and stabilize cell activity.
- **Selenium** is the key trace mineral of the vitamin E enzymes.
- **Copper** is the key trace mineral of the vitamin C enzymes.
- **Manganese** is the trace mineral which strengthens ligaments.

These are only a few examples that illustrate the role of over a hundred other minerals, all of which are equally essential.

Hydrochloric Acid

In addition to aiding in the digestion of proteins, hydrochloric acid also triggers the activity of the pancreas.

Hydrochloric acid participates in the cellular creation of electricity, one of our life forces. It helps to establish the acid-alkaline balance, which directs and controls a major part of enzyme activity. It is also responsible for solubilizing calcium and many minerals.

Water

Essential for the liquefying and absorption of nutrients, water acts as a catalyst for almost all cell biochemical reactions.

Oxygen

Like air in a fireplace or car cylinder, oxygen is necessary for all the chemical reactions of the cells.

Enzymes – the agents of life and living
(the workers and healers)

Every cell function is performed by special types of biochemical cell craftsmen called "enzymes." Enzymes are small molecules created by the DNA by combining an amino-acid (protein) with a trace mineral. Our cells may produce and use up to two hundred thousands of these active enzyme agents. Enzymes act only on bonds that connect atoms and molecules. Each enzyme can act only on one type of bond.

Enzymes have two functions: splitting molecules or combining molecules. When the chemical environment is acid, enzymes split molecules. Molecule splitting is the same as the fission processes described earlier. When the environment is alkaline the enzymes link molecules together.

During normal functions of body activity and daytime living—those times when the body needs and uses lots of energy—the body environment is generally acid; the enzymes create fission and life. During nighttime and sleep, the body environment becomes more alkaline. This is the time when enzymes link and bind molecules together, creating new substances and cells. It is also the time when the body repairs, restores and heals itself.

Enzymes are stored in cell structures called "lysosomes." Lysosomes release the exact number and type of enzymes our cells require for normal function.

When cells become damaged or worn out and their life cycle is finished, the membranes of the lysosomes rupture and release enzymes. In both of these conditions the enzymes digest the cell components. This is an essential activity. Up to 27 million cells die every minute. These dead cells must be disposed of efficiently or they will accumulate, congest the tissues and eventually denature our entire body.

Enzymes are fragile agents. After performing their many functions, eventually they become depleted and need to be replaced daily by eating enzyme rich foods that are alive, natural, unprocessed, uncontaminated and not overcooked.

Enzymes are slow, sluggish workers and must function as a team with activators, accelerators and catalysts. In this capacity they are able to supply nutrition, create energy and keep up with the active body's daily needs. Enzyme activators, accelerators, and catalyst elements are vitamins.

Vitamins are essential parts of the enzymes-protein-oil-mineral team. Together they are a dynamo; alone, they are unable to perform functions needed by the body. This synergistic team creates the food processor systems whereby cells can mold and form all of the materials that make up its structure, perform its myriad functions and bring about healing and restoration of well-being and dynamic energy.

The role of vitamins

Vitamins are not single, refined, processed chemical substances as we tend to believe from the labels on vitamin bottles. The number of identified vitamins is approximately

50, each of which is a complex structure. Most single vitamins are a combination of up to 10 different biochemicals which also act as teams. The absence of any one of these team members can jeopardize the functional efficiency of its main active constituent.

Vitamins play an important role when teaming with enzymes as catalysts and activators. However, as sole agents they contribute nothing to the structure, energy or function of body cells.

Although use of vitamins is a good step in the right direction for physiological therapy, as remedies for diseases they are much overrated. Like so many other popular notions about food supplementation, it is a simplistic panacea type of cookbook medicine.

Each vitamin can only enter and be used by cells if they have the exact chemical structure and shape that the cells require. *A synthetic vitamin cannot enter the cells.* It would be like trying to start your car with your house key.

Growth and development of cells into bodies
(The following concepts are conclusions from the research and discoveries of Dr. Raymond Bontemps of Switzerland.)[6]

All cells come into existence and acquire their specific nature, structure, functions, and place in our body organs through an amazing, almost miraculous process.

Every cell is the offspring of two original cells: an ovum and a sperm, which at a moment of joyous celebration, join together.

This united ovum and sperm divides into two cells. Each new cell in turn divides into two more cells. They multiply: 4, 8, 16, 32, 64, 120… and on and on, until a new person, or new life is created.

Our bodies are eventually comprised of between 7 to 70 trillion cells. The variation in numbers relates to the differences in body sizes and weights.

During embryonic growth as the first cells form a ball-like structure, they create small, cyst-like, fluid "bubbles." The clear fluid in these bubbles is made up of all the amino acids. Each amino acid vibrates at specific frequencies. These frequencies are special "messages" or "code-signals." The purpose of these messages is to code all cells of our bodies in a way that is similar to stamping a number onto each part of a motor, or a computer.

---

6 http://www.cryos.ch/en/dr-raymond-bontemps

Each cell and organ of our body has its own specific frequency vibration. All the body/cell frequencies are within the range of sound, or between 50-50,000 vibrations per second.

Each substance, whether it is oxygen, water, food, a chemical or drug, acts upon cells not because of their material presence or chemical action, but according to their specific frequency vibration.

Every chemical and every food, drug, antibiotic, pain pill, chemotherapy, radiation, even oxygen, has its specific frequency vibration. These individualized oscillations are crucial to the development, function, health and healing of our cells.

The code message impregnates each cell with its specific vibration, and "programs" that cell and all fetus cells to multiply and divide. It directs each cell to locate itself into specific cell tissue in a specific part of the body and creates the shape, form and design of the organs and body structure. The code message also shapes that person's features, which in turn creates its personal identity. It predetermines each cell to perform only specific functions in that specific organ.

Vibrations of the code message energize the body's life forces, which activate the nervous system as well as cell and tissue potentials. They also alert our immune defense mechanisms, which set to work to establish inter-cellular synchronization, biochemical balance and cell energy reserves.

When cells die, are damaged or destroyed, these code messages cause the dying cells to reproduce and create identical cells which will perform the same functions as their parent cells.

Each cell is a universal transmitter and receiver, similar to a radio station that transmits and receives programs to and from other stations and frequencies.

All of our cells are receptive to and affected by other vibrations with different frequencies. Frequencies that are slower than normal cell or body rates slow down, relax, or suppress the activities of those cells and the organs of which they are a part. Frequencies that are faster than normal body and cell rates will accelerate, activate, stimulate, and whip them into hyperactivity.

Vibrations and activities of the living organisms that surround us greatly impact all the cells and organs of our body. Excess and/or abnormal frequency suppression or hyperactivity is a cellular disease. Opposing frequency vibrations can counterbalance these abnormal, diseased rates and restore the normal vibrations harmonious to that cell and organ.

Restoration of normal frequencies also restores health and offsets disease.

It is the normal or disharmonious frequency vibrations—not chemicals— that determine health or disease.

Everything in our environment affects our body and our health. Frequencies we generate within ourselves and those that are generated by others around us—all the frequencies of our environment (what many call vibes), including drugs, chemicals, poisons and pollutants—affect the condition and wellness levels of our bodies and its cells.

This coding must persist throughout the life of the body. If or when cell "code programming" is destroyed or burned out, cells lose their ability to absorb and use the amino acids they require for living. When confronted with disease, they can no longer restore their structural needs. They lose their ability to reproduce and sustain their body functions. Body healing and restoration processes disintegrate.

The loss or destruction of cell programming codes can block curing even when implementing accurately selected therapies that would otherwise be extremely effective. The tissues and possibly the body as a whole will continue to degenerate. Chronic degenerative diseases will still take over. Efforts to restore health can produce confusion, discouragement and failure.

Factors that can destroy, neutralize, block, suppress, devitalize, or break down programming codes

Excessive and abnormal frequencies and vibrations of:

- Emotions triggered by fear, hatred, anger, jealousy, low self-image, and other negative attitudes.

- Negative mental vibrations of others with negative attitudes; mindsets arising from earlier traumatic experiences.

- Mental and physical burn-out, overwork, lifestyle excesses.

- Emotional and mental stresses, traumas, shocks.

- Nerve stimulants from pain, pressure or chemicals; those which create spastic tensions or which are sensed as irritating.

- Strong drugs, toxins, pollutants, chemicals, chemotherapy.

- Dead, processed, preserved, refined, synthetic and junk foods.

- Intake of foods whose vitality has been destroyed by high temperatures, overcooking, and micro-wave cooking (these alter the vibration frequency).

- Devitalization, demagnetization of cells/tissues.

- Deficiencies of vitamin/enzyme B-6 complexes, causing a loss or breakdown of the amino acids (the code carriers).

- Scars that overlap and compress nerve endings.

- Severe physical traumas, burns, frostbite.
- Any forces or substances that destroy the body or cause death.

Cell Nourishment – Nutrition

Each cell requires daily replenishment of specific nutrients. Only other living cells (plants, animals, fish, and birds) contain the hundreds of thousands of molecules of which our cells are made. Only Mother Nature can provide all the normal general needs of human nature and human cells.

Each of our trillions of cells knows which elements it has used up. These cells will then select from the hundreds of thousands of food cell molecules brought to them by the blood that it will need to perform its specific functions. It will also select molecules needed for cell structure, life force and optimal health. These molecules are then absorbed through the cell membranes and used as necessary.

Plant cells do not have as many elements and are not as complex as human cells. Only by providing a constant variety and supply of plant foods can the nourishment of all body cells be complete.

If biochemical cell elements are isolated from all the other elements of their cell of origin, arrive singly at the cell membranes and seek entrance, they will be unable to pass through that membrane. Cell elements that are unable to normalize the needs of cells are unacceptable. This means that even individual amino acids, vitamins, minerals, trace minerals, sugars and other refined processed foods are rejected.

We can compare the process of cell ingestion to baking a cake, building a motor or computer and leaving out several important ingredients or essential components. Place only three wheels on a car and try to drive it somewhere.

Mother Nature and her cell offspring are tyrants. Cells are dictators in their choices of what they allow into their domains. If we do not satisfy their demands 100% they will refuse to provide the benefits we seek. Satisfy these demands 100% and their generosity, rewards and benefits are more than gratifying.

Only living food can provide us with all the essential nutrients that:

- Create energy, vitality, morale, stamina for enjoying life to its fullest, and earning a good livelihood for self and family.
- Enable all cells and organs, such as normal bones and muscles, to grow and mature regularly; optimally fulfilling the roles for which they were intended and constructed.

- Sustain and balance all the physical, emotional and mental characteristics of the individual.

- Create the ability to resist all diseases, breakdowns, and aging processes.

- Regenerate body cells and reproduce normal, healthy and well-formed offspring.

Cell Nutrition Processes

As food molecules pass through the various organelles and nuclei of the cells, they are split into atoms. This split or fissure releases energy. When this happens, the foods have fulfilled their roles. After they have been used up and are devitalized, the initial food substances are eliminated as waste products.

Blood circulation provides transportation for proteins, oils, carbohydrates and sugars to the cells. All substances must gain access to the cells before the organ cells can incorporate and use them to perform their specific functions.

Each cell has its own hierarchy and maintains its identity throughout its lifetime. Cells must preserve the integrity of their nature or the very nature of our bodies will change. We will gradually cease to be ourselves. Disease is the name given to these distortions or aberrations.

All that is needed for creating harmony among those with differing viewpoints regarding health and healing is acceptance to the common language arising from understanding cell biochemistry, physiology and the patterns of healing dictated by cells needs. This knowledge of the human being and its cells with their myriad structures and function is so infinite in scope and so sophisticated and complex, there can be no justification for ignoring it.

Good rapport, mutual support, communication and harmony could replace current prejudice, ill feelings, inter-professional resentments and condemnations. Great minds and great professions could work together as a team.

Since all the various healthcare professions have a strong common denominator of interest in restoring well-being to their patients, it seems unrealistic that there should be any resentment among doctors of different professions, regardless of their beliefs. There must be a way to build a bridge across the broad chasm that separates the values of feuding professions.

Cells are like people, they have physical structures that are the result of heredity, behavior, attitudes, outlooks, emotions, habits, environment and lifestyle.

Chapter 7

The Philosophy of Complete Food

Hippocrates, a famous Greek physician, stated:
"Let food be your medicine and medicine be your food."

In order for us to really appreciate the wisdom of Hippocrates's words we must fully understand the meaning of "complete" food.

A complete food is one that has been produced by nature and synergistically blended with all of its constituents (proteins, minerals, enzymes and vitamins) intact. It has not been perverted or "de-natured" in any way. Each of these components is co-dependent on one another for their efficacy in performing the task Mother Nature instructed it to do. When any of these constituents becomes isolated from their teammates, they are no longer considered food by the body and lack the necessary credentials to be absorbed and used at a cellular level. With its innate wisdom, the body will reject this denatured food and target it for elimination.

Almost all of us have been guilty of buying into the propaganda of taking vitamin supplements, when in reality we are only purchasing more synthetic drugs. Vitamins purchased as isolates are made in a laboratory and differ completely from vitamins found in nature.

Vitamins are catalysts or accelerators for enzymes. They are found in foods that contain their respective enzymes and other teammates, without which they would be in disharmony with the body's needs.

When we buy vitamin C, what we are really getting is ascorbic acid. This is only a small part of a vitamin C molecule and contains none of the vitamin plasma. The best way to get more vitamin C is to increase the intake of foods high in vitamin C.

A number of years ago a group of scientists collaborated in a project to scientifically produce man-made sea water. Even the most powerful microscopes could not find any difference between real sea water and the replicated synthetic sea water. Only when they gave it the final test and introduced fish into the equation did they discover the difference.

In the "real" sea water the fish swam and survived, but when placed into its cloned counterpart, they quickly died. This only proved that Nature has secrets that even the Master doesn't reveal.

Chapter 8

The Immune System

Dr. Bernie Siegel M.D., an advocate for empowering patients and teaching survival behavior for enhancing their immune systems states:

> *Laughter and joy can mean a healing, life-enhancing message going to every cell in your body, whereas shame, guilt and despair can lead to destructive messages. Your emotions are chemical. It is exciting to understand that specific thoughts can create changes in the body. When you are happy, your body knows it. When you're depressed and feeling hopeless, your body also knows that. And when I refer to your body I mean your bone marrow, the lining of your blood vessels, your liver. Every organ participates in the happiness or sadness.*
>
> *Consciousness and knowledge occur at the cell membrane. We know that the happy individual has a different set of neuropeptides (hormones) circulating from those of the person who is depressed, angry or anxious. Our nervous system and other organ systems through these neuropeptides are communicating with every cell in our bodies. Our gut feelings, how we deal with life, how many white blood cells we produce, how rapidly a wound heals - all of these are linked.*[7]

Immunity is a mindset. Our health greatly affects our quality of life and the fulfillment of our dreams and goals. Overall health is a product of both our mental and physical well-being. We must protect our health as a precious gift from our creator by promoting positive thoughts in our conscious mind and practicing habits that energize and eliminate stress from our lives. It is imperative to identify our weak areas and also the motivators that inspire us to take control and live well.

Self-awareness is critical to our ability to consistently make wise choices and live healthy. Remember, our health truly is our wealth. You need good health to achieve your dreams and live the life you always wanted.

Immunity Resistance
Conventional medicine would have us believe that "immunity" consists only in the

---

[7] http://berniesiegelmd.com/

cells and organs that destroy viruses and bacteria. This would imply that these are the real threat to our health. This scientific thinking simply cannot be supported by facts. However, consistent dissemination of this fabrication rewards the perpetrators with huge profits while making absolutely no progress in improving the wellness of patients suffering from serious conditions.

A healthy body is equipped with amazing and marvelous mechanisms of self-protection and resistance against all diseases and causes of diseases—not just against viruses, pathogens and bacteria.

It is "armed to the teeth" with multiple defense systems and processes along with specialized organs, all designed to neutralize, control, break down, encapsulate, oxidize, burn up, destroy and eliminate every conceivable waste product, foreign substance, impurity, toxin, chemical and poison, along with every sick, dying, dead or abnormal cell, including cancer cells.

Immunity is the body's "castle wall" that, with all the necessary bodyguards and mechanisms, protects it from invaders and defends it against disease.

Host Resistance is the "military force" that attacks all invaders—that fights off and attempts to overcome and destroy insidious enemies of our health.

All diseases, whether chronic or degenerative, can only exist when organs of immunity, i.e., host resistance, detoxification and elimination, no longer function adequately.

In medical literature immunity is described as consisting of the organs and cells that control and destroy viruses and bacteria. This implies that these are the only real threats to our health.

However, all bacteria and viruses can only exist and flourish in bodies saturated with toxic foreign substances. When the body's defense organs are no longer capable of eliminating these harmful elements, bacteria and viruses multiply and thrive as a last ditch attempt to destroy the insidious wastes, poisons, and toxic substances.

Infectious agents are not menaces that destroy health. They are scavengers that are part of the body's resistance systems. Only when the poisons they feed on are rampant and not eliminated, do the bacteria or viruses develop into an army and become a threat. Each bacteria and virus creates and secretes its own waste products. These become another source of body poison. Secondarily they become destructive. The immune system is commonly referred to as those body parts that are geared to handle scavenger microbes: 1) white blood cells, 2) lymphatic channels and glands, and 3) the thymus gland.

However, this line of thought fails to consider all the other poisons and body wastes, chemicals, drugs, and pollutants that constantly menace our health in today's civilized world. The body has a multitude of other protective and offensive measures against these agents. It seems more logical to qualify all of these systems and agents as the body's immune and resistance system.

The question to ask in understanding immunity/resistance is not, "What is the immune system?" but, "What are all the enemies, threats and hazards to our health? Which part of the body, which organ, tissue, fluid, function or biochemical protects the body and prevents the onset of illness?"

Building host resistance with herbs

Cells are preserved, protected, maintained, controlled and constructed by special coils of biochemical molecules called "chromosomes." Chromosomes are amino acid/ trace mineral links of chains bound together into intricate and delicate coils of life. These reside in the cell's nucleons.[8] The nucleus of each cell is its house of government. The chromosomes are the members of its government (congress). Chromosomes are governing bodies of everything that constitutes the structure and function of cells.

No degeneration or chronic disease and no denaturing of any cell component or cell function occurs without a corresponding chemical denaturing and perversion of trace minerals and/or amino acids, which are the building blocks of chromosomes.

Chromosomes are the safeguards of health. They are the bulwarks against all degeneration and disease. Only when chromosomes are denatured does cancer occur. Since chromosomes are the forgers of enzymes and enzymes are the agents of cell life and all of its functions, if the cell enzymes cannot be manufactured, there can be no health or healing.

Chromosomes mold and create the amino acids/trace minerals into whatever special enzyme systems are required by the cell itself and by the body as a whole. The nourishing of chromosomes with trace minerals and amino-acids simultaneously generates vitality, healing, resistance and immunity.

From these observations, it should become evident that the constant and perfect provisions of living nutrients and herbs are vital to host resistance and immunity. Through their enzyme systems and biochemical activities, herbs become sources of health restoration. They have a great value when used as a part of healing regimes for the normalizing of degenerative diseases.

---

8   In chemistry and physics, a nucleon is one of the particles that makes up the atomic nucleus. Each atomic nucleus consists of one or more nucleons, and each atom in turn consists of a cluster of nucleons surrounded by one or more electrons. There are two known kinds of nucleon: the neutron and the proton. http://en.wikipedia.org/wiki/Nucleon

Immunity and resistance are our body forces and mechanisms which:

- Create defenses and barriers against disease; inhibit all diseases and disease causing processes.

- Neutralize, detoxify, attack and destroy all toxic substances that threaten our life, our cells and our bodies.

- Flush out and eliminate from the body, all residues, wastes, toxins, and substances hazardous to health, vitality, balance and well-being.

- Repair and heal all body inadequacies.

Which organ, tissue, biochemical substance, (i.e., vitamin, mineral, enzyme protein, carbohydrate or oil), life force, hormone, function or process does not play some sort of role in maintaining health, integrity, strength and viscosity and in defending our bodies against invaders, hazards and all causes of disease? The answer that should be apparent is:

Immunity is a total body function!

EVERY organ, tissue and biochemical helps in some way to: 1) protect the body and its health, or 2) resist and help fight off disease. By building the *whole* body and maintaining *every* biochemical and function, we create immunity and resistance to all disease.

Immunity is not just the activity of any one organ, immune body, blood cell, or biochemical.

The building and maintaining of total health is a function of enzymes, controlled and governed by healthy chromosomes and balanced by hormones. Throughout our bodies are hundreds of thousands of enzymes.

The key factors of immunity and resistance responsible for every aspect of healing and for every single life function are enzymes.

Without an understanding of enzymes, very little of the science of herbal healing can be appreciated and properly utilized. Possibly the most important service this book can provide is to clarify the enzymatic nature of herbs and the nature and functions of enzymes.

Chapter 9

Enzymes

Enzymes are the agents, executors, and creators
of all functions: healing, life and living.

**Enzymes are microscopic molecules of amino acids
(proteins) and trace minerals that are linked together.**

Each enzyme has only one specific function and performs only one specific action. That action is entirely dependent on the pH balance of the environment. When the environment of cells or tissues in which they work is acid, the enzymes split molecules and when the environment is alkaline, the same enzymes link together the same molecules that they separate in the acid environment.

During the daytime our bodies are acid. The splitting of molecules in this environment produces fission resulting in the production and release of energy. This energy is used for daily activities and functions. At night when sleeping, our bodies and cell environments become alkaline. In an alkaline environment, enzymes link together the same molecules that they separate in an acid environment. The joining of molecules creates new substances and cells. This is the process of body healing and restoration. However, if only one necessary component is missing, the process cannot be completed and repair does not take place.

The roles and functions of enzymes

Enzymes are wonder workers; they are the body's artisans and craftsmen. Enzyme systems are the most valuable and effective agents for restoring, maintaining and regenerating cells and our body's immunity and host resistance.

Enzymes are the life of our bodies, as well as the foods by which they are manufactured. They are the forces that activate virtually every biochemical process that occurs in our bodies. Enzymes perform every activity and ALL the functions of living. Without enzymes, life itself does not and cannot exist. They are responsible for our thinking, feeling, talking, and seeing.

Enzymes are carpenters

Enzymes build the structures of all cells. They serve as catalysts for activating and accomplishing the restoration and normalization of body chemistry. No effective or complete health restoration can occur without the presence and action of the essential enzymes and enzyme systems naturally found in the body.

To maintain normalcy and balance of all body structures and functions, hundreds of thousands of these normalizing, healing, restoring, biochemical protecting miracle workers must be functioning 24/7—day and night.

Enzymes are our body's healing experts

Enzymes are healers in action. The words "heal" and "health," are derived from ethnic words meaning "whole." When a being is in a state of wholeness, everything required for its perfection is present, normal and in balance. Nothing is lacking. To heal is to make whole—to make everything whole.

Some enzymes are demolition experts

Demolition enzymes destroy old dead cells and cell debris and eliminate them from our bodies. Some of these demolition agents are our digestive enzymes. These enzymes break down and fragment foods, sick cells, dying cells, foreign cells, and abnormal cells, even cancer cells. They digest the fragments and debris that are the leftovers of cell breakdown. They also digest all foreign substances whose chemical constituents are similar to our cellular chromosomes. (Bacteria, viruses and fungi have identical biochemical compositions as chromosomes.) Amazingly, digestive enzymes do not attack healthy cells and normal body biochemicals.

All cells are made up of similar substances. The bonds that hold together the molecules of plant and animal cells are similar to those of human cells. Only the arrangements of the molecules in the cell structures differ.

The enzymes required to break down our body cells are the same as those required for the digestion of our foods. Our digestive enzymes can break down all foods, regardless of their cell composition. They perform equally well on both human and food cells.

Our digestive enzymes, those secreted mainly by the pancreas, do not die or disappear into thin air after they have performed their function, nor do they undergo a chemical change. After meals, they pass with foods into our bloodstream and penetrate every cell of our bodies.

These intelligent agents search out and destroy all abnormal, denatured, tired, dying cells and fragment them into molecules. They change the residue of these cells into forms that can readily be flushed out and eliminated from the body.

Digestion takes place in every square inch of our bodies. Every cell is made up of hundreds of thousands of biochemical molecules. Up to 27 million cells die every minute (2-3 billion a day). It requires an enormous army of enzymes to process and disintegrate these trillions of molecular structures and transform them into substances that can readily be eliminated or converted into other substances that our bodies then recycles.

We would not live very long if the dead cell debris and waste were not flushed from our systems. This waste has to be completely digested or it would accumulate in our tissues. In the process of rotting, it would eventually pollute our entire body.

If cancer cells, microbes, viruses, and similar substances survive in our systems, it has to mean, in addition to other reasons, that the amounts and types of enzymes that our bodies use to control and destroy them are insufficient.

Dead cells are like cadavers. They need to be broken down and eliminated or they will accumulate in our tissues and poison us. In every cell are special enzymes. They are stored in cell organelles called "lysosomes." The lysosome membranes rupture and release their enzymes, which auto-digest all the cell components. This is the same process that makes all foods rot, turn into compost, and return to the soil when left in a field. These are referred to as metabolic enzymes and work inside the cells. Digestive enzymes work outside the cell.

If the metabolic enzymes in cells are absent, auto-digestion of those cells can be blocked. It may become difficult for the body and its external digestive enzymes to properly deal with these cells.

External cell digesting enzymes are unable to destroy cells while acting alone. They work in conjunction with and need the action of similar metabolic enzymes in the cells.

One reason why it may be so difficult to deal with cancer cells is the fact that they lack cell digesting enzymes. In their absence, the cancer cells remain unusually hardy, resistant to fragmentation and difficult to get rid of.

Is it possible that herbs can provide the missing enzymes, making it possible to successfully destroy cancer cells?

Enzymes are detoxifiers

Some enzymes have an affinity for every type of chemical. They react and combine with abnormal and poisonous substances and render them harmless. These enzymes also bind neutral molecules to the harmful ones. In so doing, they change the nature of toxins, chemicals and poisons, thereby rendering them increasingly less toxic and thus, more harmless. They split off harmful, toxic molecules from a poisonous substance and fragment them. This process also renders them into a harmless non-toxic state.

An unhealthy lifestyle can introduce toxins into our bodies faster than the detoxification process can eliminate them. This is why lifestyle changes are also a necessary part of good health.

Detoxification is the process of enzymatic neutralizing and breaking down of toxins and poisons, and the flushing out of ALL body wastes—all excesses, toxins, poisons, and chemicals.

Enzymes neutralize and destroy toxins, body wastes, poisons, even carcinogens that circulate through the blood as they are being channeled to the liver for detoxification. When they reach the liver they are broken down into molecular forms that can readily be eliminated.

The main organ of our body responsible for these functions is our liver. Our livers are laboratories of enzymes. The hundreds of thousands of enzymes that work in the healthy liver are capable of performing biochemical tasks that would require a fully equipped, completely staffed laboratory the size of a large city.

To summarize, enzymes are the principle agents of our many organs and systems of detoxification and elimination.

Failure to detoxify:
- Leaves substances in the body that can persist in causing disease.
- Allows toxins to continue to undermine immunity.
- Encourages intense breakdown of enzymes.
- Overloads liver and organs of detoxification and elimination.
- Seriously depletes life and healing forces.

Enzymes are the natural, active factors inside white blood cells. These cells act as scavengers and destroyers of blood toxins.

Enzymes work in teams with hormones and antibodies
Enzymes are the major agent that our cells use to create hormones and antibodies.

Enzymes act only as members of a special biological team. Regardless of the importance of their roles, they are unable to function without the assistance and teamwork of other biochemicals.

Each component of this team functions together as a unit. Individually they are ineffective. Each is indispensable to the total function of the whole team.

Absence of even a single enzyme weakens our ability to mobilize resistance to disease.

The personality of enzymes

Enzymes are slow, sluggish workers. By themselves, they are incapable of keeping up with the body's need for fuel, energies and body structural material. They cannot bring about all the changes and supply all the body's needs as rapidly as our daily lifestyle requires. They need a catalyst, something that speeds up their action. Enzymes only function and work in teams with their accelerators. The activators/accelerators of enzymes are vitamins and minerals.

Nature's enzyme factories

No drug company or laboratory is capable of manufacturing these active living biochemical components, yet every living cell on the planet creates them by the tens of thousands.

Every one of the 70 trillion human cells along with the cells of animals, fish, birds, trees and flowers are enzyme factories. Every cell contains an enzyme "design and production room."

The amount and kind of enzymes manufactured by each cell is limited to the amounts of proteins and trace minerals they can obtain from the food we eat.

Each plant has a natural affinity for specific minerals and trace minerals. By breaking down the soil waters which the root absorbs, the plant obtains hydrogen and oxygen. It also absorbs nitrogen and oxygen from the air. The plant links nitrogen with the hydrogen to form amino acids.

These plants (enzyme factories) that produce specific enzymes for healing specific ailments and also for maintaining optimal health, are known as "herbs."

In chapter 16, after presenting more information about the various body organs and systems and how they function, we will discuss the extraordinary power of whole food herbs as cleansing and detoxing agents, nutritional supplements, and body builders.

Chapter 10

Proteins

The Importance of Quality Proteins

Proteins are the building blocks of all body cells and tissues. They provide the foundation for life itself. As the most essential elements for the structure, life forces, fluids, organs, glands, and healing processes of every cell, organ and tissue of the human body, proteins are necessary for every aspect of living.

Without quality proteins there is no health, function, individuality, blood, feeling, thinking or being. More important than vitamin or mineral deficiencies is a health regime that is rich and balanced with proteins.

Anything that interferes with cellular supply of required amino acids contributes to the degeneration, death or abnormal growth of both cells and organs. Almost all diseases, degeneration, deterioration, denaturing, imbalance, and body function—even the body's inability to digest, absorb, and fully utilize protein molecules—are in some way related to protein deficiency.

The word "protein" means *first*. After air and water, proteins are the first and most necessary foods. A quality protein diet and efficient body use of proteins are the first aspects to be considered and maintained for any good health program. Understanding proteins and learning how to use them is one of the most essential aspects in maintaining and restoring health.

It is essential to learn as much as you can about the whole picture of proteins so the ideas and recommendations included in this book become a permanent and important part of your daily lifestyle. This knowledge could prove to be one of the most valuable assets of your entire health program.

Protein foods are considered "quality" or "complete" when they consist of almost all of the 26 amino acids and 8 essential ones—and when the proportions of each of the essential amino acids is adequate to provide all the body's needs.

The *balance* of amino acids in a food is just as critical as the *amounts*. The value of any protein food is determined by the individual's need for the specific amino acids it contains.

No food is biochemically constructed so that all of its nutrients correspond completely to the body's biochemistry; nor does it contain nutrients in identical proportion to those of the human body. Animal foods come close to being similar in composition. Plant foods are not formulated like human cells.

Proteins are not unchanging substances, fixed and deposited for a lifetime. They are in a constant state of change and exchange. Their molecules are constantly being broken down and worn-out, requiring replacement.

Each protein food provides the basic nutrients for structure and function of body cells and cell organs (organelles). Protein foods nourish the genes and chromosomes that dominate cell integrity, growth and function.

Every disease, illness, or abnormality in the body is related in some way to proteins!

Health challenges related to protein deficiencies:

- Atrophy of any and all organs and tissues of the body.

- Imbalance and inadequate functioning of any of the endocrine glands.

- Premature aging, degeneration and atrophy of the skin (wrinkles, folds and skin diseases).

- Thinning and loss of hair, baldness.

NOTE: The conditions of skin, hair and finger nails are excellent measures of protein levels and availability. Brittleness and fragility invariably indicate a lack of proteins.

- Edema – upset body fluid balances, causing swelling of feet, legs, and area around the eyes; abnormal fluid retention.

- Poor and slow healing of wounds, bruises, cuts, etc.

- Anemia; loss of red or white blood cells.

- Loss of/or shrinking of muscles and ligaments, with loosening, slipping and clicking of joints.

- Bone degeneration - osteoporosis, and/or arthritis.

- Habitual and general weakness and/or fatigue.

- Sensitivity to the cold.

- High blood pressure.
- Nervousness, irritability, mental and emotional instability.
- Apathy, loss of enthusiasm and enjoyment of living.
- Degeneration of the liver. This organ suffers more than any other from protein deficiencies. Many of its multiple functions break down, allowing toxic substances to accumulate. Resistance to disease and normal healing are markedly weakened.
- Symptoms of starvation, even when all the other nutrients needed by the body are in plentiful supply.
- Constipation due to flabby conditions of the intestinal muscles.
- Weight loss, stunted growth, emaciation.

Protein deficiencies lead to:
- Arthritis, cavities, poor teeth, poor ligaments, with tendencies to dislocations, sprains, and hernias.
- Personality changes: loss of ambition, drive, enthusiasm and joy of living.
- Depressive, lethargic, demoralizing exhaustion. Energy is as important to the brain as it is to muscles and every other organ of the body.
- Skin problems: itching, skin eruptions, acne, boils.
- Toxic states: Almost all degenerative diseases have some form of toxicity.

All protein deficiency breakdowns and changes that affect the body are reversible by adequately replenishing total body protein needs.

A deficiency, however slight or brief, can render the body more prone to disease. Acute deficiencies can be life threatening.

A meal without quality proteins is a meal that allows the onset of deficiency, starvation and a weakening of the body structures and functions.

Protein intake is not simply a matter of including meat, (soy) beans, lentils or a similar high concentrate protein in your daily diet. Balancing protein intake is an art.

OBTAINING, USING AND BALANCING QUALITY PROTEINS

You are eating a "Disease Diet" if:
- You don't buy wholesome food.
- You don't prepare food properly.
- You don't digest and assimilate it properly.

No one, not even expert nutritionists, succeeds in maintaining meals of quality balance without giving careful consideration to the protein foods selected in the preparation of each meal. It is important to remember that practically all foods contain some protein.

Proteins are the structural materials of the cells of all plants, animals and humans. Every time you eat a solid food, regardless of whether that food is listed as a "high protein" food, you are getting some needed amino acids.

Nature never provides isolated proteins. All natural foods contain complexes of proteins.

Diet Variety

By eating a variety of foods you will satisfy all body and health needs. The body can only obtain sufficient quality proteins if it is provided with a variety of protein foods, from which it takes what it needs as it needs it.

Meat foods provide proportions similar to body needs, but meat amino acids are considerably more difficult for the body to use than those of vegetables. Meats contain higher concentrations of proteins.

Vegetable proteins have much simpler molecular structures and thus are more easily digested and used by the body. A vegetable diet can easily provide all the proteins required for health; however, the vegetables must be living. They cannot be denatured or destroyed by cooking. Excess cooking can destroy up to 90% of plant proteins and their enzymes.

People eating overcooked meals should include meat in their diet so the amount of proteins left over after heat destruction may better supply sorely needed proteins.

Foods contain amino acids in hundreds of different combinations.

Amino acid proportions are maintained only by food intake containing complete proteins at each meal, either in one food or in a combination of foods that provide all the essential amino acids.

Protein amounts required for health

The average body burns up or uses approximately 2 ounces (about 60 grams) of protein daily. At least this much protein must be replenished daily, plus an extra amount to provide for body maintenance and unexpected needs, e.g., increased exercise, stresses, overwork, etc.

Proteins cannot be stored and must be replenished daily. Every cell stores the proteins it needs, but the body does not store extra reserves of proteins for future use. Whatever is not needed at that time is turned into energy reserves or foods. Pregnancy markedly increases a mother's protein requirements.

Inadequate intake of proteins causes the body to mobilize and use proteins from other regions. Protein starved tissues will absorb amino acids from the muscles—and even from the stomach and intestinal cells. This depletion can cause stomach ulcers.

With age, although most people's diets decrease in protein intake, the body's protein needs increase. Aging cells die quicker and are damaged easier as they are affected by life's traumas and stresses.

As the body ages, it becomes a greater challenge to provide adequate protein in balanced proportions.

A raw (or undercooked) vegetable diet together with moderate portions of either high quality or quantity protein foods listed at the end of this chapter, provide more than enough protein for the ordinary demands of daily living.

It is possible to eat too much protein or more than the body can utilize or burn up during its daily activities. A large meat intake or more than one meal of meat per day will not normally be used up by the body except by those living a strenuous or physically active life (sports, physical labor, overwork, etc.).

Excess proteins require excess activity of the body organs, including the stomach, pancreas, liver, heart, kidneys, and intestines. Overworking any organ eventually depletes its reserves, making it conducive to eventual illness.

Protein metabolism (body use)

All proteins must be broken down into free or individual amino acids before they can be used by the body. Each amino acid is joined to others by means of "couplings." Each type of amino acid coupling requires its own specific enzyme to split it.

The first stage of this process is digestion. Stomach acids and enzymes initiate the breakdown of complex amino acid combinations. Pancreatic enzymes complete this process and transform the amino acids into a state in which they can be absorbed through the intestines and enter the liver.

Upon exiting the liver they are then carried by the blood to different tissues and reassembled into the special combinations that make up the proteins to: 1) replace cell material that has worn out, 2) add to tissue that needs to grow, and 3) make enzymes or hormones and other necessary active compounds required by the body.

This process is absolutely precise and operates on an "all or none" principle. If the body cannot build a complete protein from the nutrients it was given, no activity will occur.

Supplementing protein needs

In cases of prolonged and serious body depletion of proteins, it may be imperative to replenish body needs with a protein supplement or concentrate. Diet alone may not be capable of catching up with long term and serious body deficiency. This is especially true in cases of degenerative diseases or diseases involving abnormal growth, such as cancer or inadequate healing patterns that often come with aging.

The body can absorb and utilize only so many nutrients from the diet in a single day. If a supplement is to be used, it must be in a natural, organic and unprocessed "food concentrate" form. Any substitute is unsatisfactory, possibly even detrimental.

The process of concentrating proteins must not involve the destruction or extraction of any of nature's accompanying elements, especially its enzymes. It must not involve heat, chemicals, or any other process that may denature the amino acids. Unfortunately, many protein concentrates, even those sold by health stores and vitamin companies, do not comply with these requisites. Often they include hydrolyses and pre-digested proteins. Please avoid using these products.

Quality protein food list:

Almonds, Hazelnuts, Peanuts, Coconut, Brewer's Yeast, Bone Marrow, Sunflower Seeds, Wheat grass, Brown Rice, Sesame Seeds, Potatoes, Flax Seeds, Avocadoes, Soybeans, Bananas, Eggs, Carob (powder), Sprouts (all kinds), Mushrooms, Mixed Raw Vegetables, Peanut Butter, Walnuts, Spirulina, Kelp, Dulse.

These foods also contain smaller amounts of quality proteins:

Asparagus, Carrots, Other Nuts, Buckwheat, Alfalfa, Beets, Broccoli, Peas, Cauliflower, Eggplant, Squash, Wheat Germ (vacuum packed, freezer stored).

NOTE: The above are the advisable, protein foods which contain a complete and balanced quota and variety of essential amino acids.

Each meal should contain at least one of the proteins from the high quality foods list. Particular importance should be placed on eating a quality protein at breakfast: one of the nuts, eggs, sesame seeds, flax seeds, coconuts, or other quality food of your choice.

Chapter 11

Minerals

Although most Americans take in plenty of calories,
their mineral intake is drastically deficient.

Keep it in balance

The human body is complex and requires both minerals and trace minerals to maintain health. In order to do so, however, these minerals and nutrients **must exist in balance.** As researchers have continued to conduct more human health studies, the relationship between a balanced ratio of minerals and health levels has become increasingly evident.

Maintaining balance becomes complex because body processes are constantly using mineral nutrients that must be renewed regularly. This is only possible by eating a diet rich in minerals—the right ones, in balance. Although most Americans take in plenty of calories, their mineral intake is drastically deficient. In fact, an estimated 90% of Americans suffer a mineral deficiency or imbalance.

The human health industry's approach to balance has not curtailed the problem. When a study highlights the importance of a particular mineral, the industry responds by providing that single nutrient in isolation. This is unfortunate, since the studies also point out inadequacies of this approach.

Although most doctors and therapists recognize the necessity for the body to have certain minerals to accomplish its work and preserve its health, only a few realize these minerals must be in their organic state for the body to accept and utilize them.

Understanding the facts
- Minerals are inorganic if they exist naturally in the soil and water.
- Minerals are organic if they exist in plants and animals.
- Only plants can transform inorganic minerals into organic minerals.

- Animals must eat plants or plant-eating animals to obtain their organic minerals.

- Inorganic minerals are useless and injurious to the animal organism.

How the confusion began

Early nutritionists did not distinguish between inorganic and organic minerals because both have the same chemical compositions. The mineral iron in the bloodstream has the same chemical composition as the mineral iron in a nail—iron is iron, after all. However, these nutritionists incorrectly reasoned that there were no other differences between these two forms of iron. Consequently, they actually produced iron mineral supplements that consisted of surplus powdered nails.

Perhaps you've heard the expression, "Mad enough to chew nails." In this case, mad or unbalanced is certainly the correct word.

These nutritionists wrongly assumed that a chemical similarity in minerals also meant there was a nutritive similarity between organic and inorganic minerals. Although it is true that the same minerals found in the human body are also found in the soil and water, it is incorrect to assume that the minerals in the soil are food for man. We are not soil eaters; we are plant eaters.

It is necessary that minerals in the soil be elaborated into organic compounds by the plant before they can be assimilated by the body. The various mineral compounds produced by the chemist differ in structure and relative positions of their component molecules from those produced in the plant.

Over sixty years ago a German scientist named Abderhalden conducted a series of experiments comparing the way several species absorbed different forms of iron. He found that animals fed with food that had inadequate amounts of organic iron in addition to inorganic iron were unable in the long run to produce as much hemoglobin as those receiving a natural or organic iron-sufficient diet.

Although the inorganic iron may be absorbed into the body, it is not utilized in the formation of hemoglobin, but remains unused within the tissues. Abderhalden also concluded that any apparent benefit of the inorganic iron resulted from its stimulating effect.

Chemically it is true that iron in the bloodstream and iron in nails are the same, and calcium in rocks (known as dolomite) is identical to calcium in the bones.

However, it is a grave error to believe the body can digest, assimilate and utilize powdered nails and crushed rocks.

Mineral Supplements

The idea of administering inorganic minerals as foods and remedies for man started with the German scientist, Hensel, in the early twentieth century. Later, homeopaths expanded his idea and made numerous artificial mineral preparations called cell salts, which are still sold today as popular "cures" for mineral deficiencies. Today mineral supplements exist in many forms and come from many sources. They are all useless. Mineral supplements are of no benefit to the body if they are either inorganic or isolates. If mineral supplements are inorganic, the body cells cannot use them. In fact, the body must work harder to compensate for and eliminate the waste created by ingesting these supplements. The body accelerates its eliminative activities and works hard to expel these foreign substances. This stimulation is often mistaken for the "beneficial action" of the supplement. Actually, the supplements are not beneficial—*they are very harmful.* They are inanimate and toxic.

As health consumers have grown more educated in the differences between organic and inorganic minerals, so have producers of these supplements. Consequently, there are now mineral supplements which are advertised as coming from "organic" sources. These products are equally harmful/ineffective because the minerals exist in an isolated state, removed and separated from their natural teammates—vitamins, enzymes, minerals, proteins, etc.—that accompany them in their natural source and synergistically provide them with their crucial life energy vibrations.

Minerals must be consumed in their natural, un-isolated and organic state to be of any use to the body. The best mineral supplements are those naturally occurring in complete or whole mineral-rich, unprocessed foods.

Mineral Waters

Mineral waters cannot provide any beneficial minerals to the body. All minerals contained in such waters are inorganic and will be targeted for elimination by the body. Should an excess of these inorganic minerals be consumed in the water, the body cannot rid itself of them fast enough and they are deposited in the body.

These inorganic mineral deposits lead to kidney and gallstone formation, hardening of the arteries, premature aging, heart trouble, ossification of the brain and other serious diseases. Waste mineral matter from mineral-containing waters combines with cholesterol to form multiple plaques. These plaques lead to cardiovascular problems and join with uric acid to cause gout, arthritis, rheumatism and other inflammatory challenges.

Body cells reject all inorganic minerals consumed in mineral-laden waters.

When mineralized waters are consumed, a condition known as "leukocytosis" occurs within the body thirty minutes to three hours after drinking. Leukocytosis is the proliferation of white blood cells, which are the body's first line of defense against foreign and harmful body substances. Thus, the inorganic minerals in the water are the catalyst for leukocytosis to occur, and as such, unable to provide the first line of defense.

Mineral waters cannot furnish the body with any necessary elements other than the water itself. The remaining inorganic minerals are either eliminated through the skin, kidneys, etc., or they are deposited within the body where they may cause eventual harm.

Sea water is our richest mineral water, yet it is toxic to the body. Similarly, all other mineralized waters are simply dirty waters, contaminated with inorganic matter that is pathogenic to the body.

How Inorganic Minerals are Transformed

Even plants in their embryonic state cannot use inorganic minerals in the soil, but instead feed on the organic compounds contained within its seed. Not until its roots and leaves are grown can a plant utilize the inorganic minerals of the soil.

The transformation of inorganic into organic matter takes place principally in the green leaves of the plant by means of photosynthesis. Only by the presence of chlorophyll is the plant able to utilize the inorganic carbon molecule and convert it with hydrogen and oxygen into organic combinations of starch and sugar. Ultimately, the plant combines nitrogen and other mineral elements from the soil into more complex organic combinations. Only chlorophyll-bearing plants have the ability to assimilate iron, calcium and other minerals from the soil and use the resulting combinations to construct nucleo-proteins.

Vital changes occur in all minerals as they pass from the soil into the structure of plants. These changes created by the magic of nature cannot be replicated by any mechanical, chemical or human processes. Attempting to do so would be somewhat akin to the old medical practice of dissecting cadavers to look for evidence of the human soul.

Minerals and Human Health

A significant body of evidence points to the fact that minerals by themselves and in proper balance to one another have important biochemical and nutritional functions. To understand the concept of "biochemical individuality" we have to discard the mistaken assumption that every person utilizes and absorbs minerals the same way.

The absorption of minerals is dependent on so many different factors, not the least of which are age, adequacy of stomach acid output, balanced bowel flora, lack of intestinal illnesses and parasites, and dietary fiber intake.

Regardless of the nutritional potential of a food, its contribution is nonexistent if it does not pass the test of absorption first through the gut wall and then into the cell. The nutrients from the organism's environment that have been made available by absorption are then transported through the circulatory system to the cells, where they serve their ultimate purpose upon which all life depends, viz., participation in cellular metabolic activities.

Chapter 12

Acid-Alkaline Balance & Health

In health and healing, acid/alkaline balance is
among the most essential to maintain.

Acids and alkalines determine the very nature of our body biochemicals and the quality of each body function. They manipulate the disposition of all body biochemical structures and activities. They also provide the fertile soil in which our life forces take shape and flourish, and the biochemical conditions required for rebuilding, repairing, and restoring cells. Acids and alkalines create the conditions by which our energies are created for our daily activities.

In a biochemical environment of acidity or alkalinity, all foods travel to the cells for which they are destined. No food, medication or drug can be used by the body metabolism in a beneficial way if the biochemical terrain of the body is not in a proper acid-alkaline balance.

The acid-alkaline balance is both the foundation and starting point for body health and healing. This balance is critical for determining the environment in which all enzymes act, and also for recognizing that *all* healing results from the activity of enzymes.

Healing involves the sum total of all body acids, alkalines, proteins, minerals and enzymes. Any acid or alkaline excess can seriously impede healing processes.

Clearing out body wastes, poisons and toxic cell debris is the first step toward creating conditions favorable for healing.

Acids – Alkalines & Enzymes

Enzymes, as discussed in Chapter 9, are microscopic molecules consisting of the union of a trace mineral with a particle of a protein called an "amino acid." Each of the possibly four to five hundreds of thousands of enzymes performs only one function. They manipulate the chemical bonds that hold together all molecules and substances. These bonds are like the links of a chain.

Enzymes act in only one of two ways. Either they break the links between molecules or they create links that bind molecules together.

Enzymes are the core of life and living. Our enzymes are the tools, workmen and agents responsible for every aspect of our living—for every function of our organs, every hormone, nutrient and substance in our bodies. Enzymes create our energies and life forces. They also neutralize and fight off all pollutants that threaten to poison our body and its environment. Without our huge army of enzymes we could not perform any of the life functions.

Although all healing in the body is the result of the biochemical activity of enzymes, these agents are totally dependent on the environment of acids and alkalines in which they perform. A body that is excessively acid is excessively stimulated and active. Energy reserves become depleted. Exhaustion is inevitable. A body doesn't heal when it is active and burning up large amounts of energy.

In order to promote cell growth, rebuild and restore heath, the body has to slow down, relax, stop and shift gears from an acid to an alkaline state.

When the body environment shifts from acid to alkaline, the same enzymes reverse their role. Instead of separating molecules to make energy, they now link molecules together. During this process they build new biochemicals, cells and tissue in a way that is similar to putting together the pieces of a gigantic jig-saw puzzle.

Knowledge about body acidity and alkalinity and biochemical balance is basic to understanding the dynamics of health and healing.

The daily acid-alkaline shift

Our bodies alternate from alkalinity to acidity during the day and the reverse during the night. Daily activities and the problems and stresses of living gradually use up energy resources created for that day.

The body must be alkaline in order for cell replacement and repair to occur. Cell protoplasm is high in potassium, the most alkaline of minerals. Cells that have burned out become fragmented and are destroyed. When they die, the cells dump their protoplasm and potassium into the body biochemical pool. Our body biochemistry gradually shifts to the alkaline side.

When body fluids are acid, enzymes split the bonds that link molecules. This molecular fission is similar to an atomic explosion. Fission creates energy. Molecular fission provides the life force energies required to perform our daily activities.

All body activities, work, exercise and forms of stress, including mental and emotional activities, depend on a healthy body metabolism. Excesses in any of these areas increase the rate of metabolism, breakdown of cells and build-up of body wastes and alkalines.

Billions of cells wear out and die daily. Their cell sacs (membranes) collapse, liberating their mineral content. As mentioned earlier, cell protoplasm is rich in potassium. Of all the minerals, it is the most alkaline. The greater and more intense the activity, stress, wear and tear, the greater the cell disintegration and their release of potassium. Potassium levels accumulate in the body fluids. This causes the body's alkaline levels (alkalosis) to gradually increase.

Potassium has possibly the greatest influence on cells and their environment. As the alkaline resources increase, the enzymes switch their activities from producing energy to rebuilding the body and its cells. The body slows down; it experiences fatigue and starts to relax. The muscle cells lose their energy (acidity). It is time for sleep. The importance of potassium intake cannot be underestimated.

Body chemistries that stay acid remain constantly in a state of accelerated metabolism. The result is exhaustion and burn-out. Energies caused by cell fission continue to stimulate and activate our body systems. We keep going… and going until all our reserves are depleted.

When acidity is excessive, our bodies shift into a state of acidosis which can manifest itself in a number of different ways such as: hypersensitivities, irritability, nervousness, insomnia, restlessness, disturbed sleep and over-reacting.

Factors that increase body acidity

Excessive physical, mental and emotional activities, stresses and tensions, increase the metabolism rate, which in turn increases the demand on our mineral supply, often to the point of depletion. When this happens, minerals pour out of our bodies and through our kidneys like salt pouring through a sieve.

The adrenal or anti-stress gland controls and operates the body's mineral supplies, giving it what it needs in order to perform its activities, whether minimal, moderate or excessive. If activities are excessive over a period of time, extreme alkaline loss is inevitable. This can be very detrimental. Over-sweating will also cause an excessive loss of sodium, releasing many of the same alkaline minerals through the skin.

In the processes of repairing and healing, our bodies use up alkaline reserves and return the body to an acid state.

As cells grow, multiply and divide while replacing and creating new cells, they absorb potassium.

Acid Diets

The average western world diet consists of great excesses of acid foods. For most people, 90% of their food is acid in nature.

Acid foods include all:

- Grains, cereals, and seeds.
- Foods made from grains and flours.
- Nuts, oils, fats, butter, and margarines.
- High concentrate protein foods: meats, fish.
- Some fruits and their juices: prunes, cranberries, and plums.
- Wines and alcoholic beverages.
- Sugar foods, sweets, and desserts.
- Vinegars and fermented foods, e.g., sauerkraut.
- All junk foods: hamburgers, hot dogs, barbecues, ice creams, sandwiches, sweets, and candies.
- Soft drinks; they contain so much acid, if all the acids in one normal can or bottle were absorbed, it might take a month for our bodies to metabolize and use them.
- Most vitamin pills, e.g., ascorbic acid and pantothenic acid.
- All oil soluble vitamins: A, D E and F.
- Excessive use of acid-type tablets, e.g., hydrochloric acid, acetyl salicylic acid (aspirin), antibiotics.

When alkalinity is excessive our bodies shift into a state of alkalosis.

Alkalosis manifests itself in the following ways:

- Extreme fatigue, feelings of lethargy, sluggishness.
- Loss of ambition and initiative.
- Feelings of inadequacy.
- Faulty digestion, burning in the stomach, intestinal gas, bloating, fatigue, sleepiness after meals.

Factors that increase alkalinity

Without the condition of alkalinity, cells cannot repair or rebuild. Healing and restoration to health and well-being cannot occur. Alkalinity levels gradually build up and replace acidity of the blood and body fluids, causing us to feel sleepy.

Sleep is a state of alkalinity. The metabolism slows down and healing takes place. Enzymes help the cells rebuild by reconnecting instead of splitting their molecules.

During sleep time all restoration, repairing, healing and rebuilding of our bodies takes place.

Eating a meal causes a temporary increase of alkalinity. Food that passes through the stomach triggers the secretion and release of hydrochloric acid. This acid solubilizes and releases the alkaline minerals and substances of foods. Until these alkalize and nutrients are used up by the body, their presence will increase overall body alkalinity.

An excess of alkaline and alkalizing foods can accumulate and influence body alkalinity. Protein rich foods, vegetables and fruits have this action.

Of all foods, only fruits and vegetables are alkaline. Therefore, they must form the basis of our daily intake of nutrients.

Fruits and vegetables, not meat and potatoes, are the foundations for body nourishment and balance.

Tums, Maalox, Mylanta, and numerous other antacids neutralize hydrochloric acid as well as other body acids from the stomach. This neutralization process can destroy our energies and life force reserves.

Even a slight variation in pH[9] creates distresses and diseases. Any excess or deficiency of essential acids or alkalines can seriously affect health and block the healing effects of therapies, regimes, diets or supplements.

The body metabolism cannot use foods, medications and healing supplements unless the chemical environment of the body is in normal "acid-alkaline" balance. When the pH balance is not taken into consideration and its imbalance blocks healing, too often we end up believing that certain disease conditions are incurable. Most of us innocently live a "suicidal" type of living because we don't realize that all acid and alkaline excesses affect our inner biochemical world.

In the Appendix is a list of acid- and alkaline- forming foods, respectively.

Consequence and side effects of acid-alkaline imbalances

The blood is a tyrant. It demands absolute, constant and perfect acid-alkaline balance and will not tolerate any deviation from normal. Since the blood transports every nutrient that travels to the cells, it follows that each of these nutrients must be in harmonious pH balance with the blood. All substances of different pH automatically react with each other. The nature of each is changed.

---

9 The term used in chemistry to measure acid-alkaline balance

Foods that contact a chemical environment that is in contrast, either too acid or too alkaline, will undergo a chemical reaction and change. They will be denatured and will no longer be of nutritional value to the cells, nor supply what the cells require to sustain their energies, life force, or structural integrity.

It takes many years to deplete the body of either its acid or alkaline reserves. It can also take a long time to restore the normal body acid-alkaline balance that has been disrupted by years of excesses, abuses, and losses.

Aging is commonly associated with a decreased secretion of hydrochloric acid in the stomach. As the level of hydrochloric acid output decreases, the body's ability to digest and release minerals from food intake diminishes. Inability to adequately absorb these minerals may be one of the causes of age-associated degeneration. For this reason, it is important to pay careful attention to those factors that will assist in maintaining adequate hydrochloric acid levels.

Chapter 13

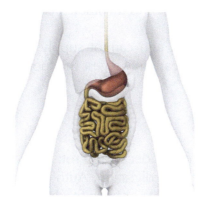

Stomach Health (Digestion)

*Digestion is the preparation of foods for replenishing
all of our daily nutritional needs.*

Stomach Health

Many people nonchalantly treat their digestion as a type of garbage pail into which they can dump anything that pleases their palate or titillates their taste buds. They tend to believe that as long as they experience no immediate discomforts, pain, distress, nausea or other symptoms, this eating lifestyle is perfectly all right.

For those who wish to learn more about establishing and maintaining healthy eating habits, it is important to better appreciate the process of digestion—what actually happens to the food we eat and why it may be valuable to reconsider a lifestyle of random eating versus one that consciously ensures optimal intake of healthy food choices.

Our stomach is the starting point for all body needs. Any failure to produce and secrete all the enzymes and acids essential for digestion sets into action a whole series of dysfunctions and starts a vicious cycle of deficiencies, problems and complications.

If our digestive system does not perform as it should, every cell and function of the body will suffer. Perfect health and healing cannot occur if the stomach is unhealthy.

**Proper care and consideration of stomach health
is the first step toward optimal body health and healing.**

Digestion is the process by which the stomach breaks down foods into its nutrient molecules. Enzymes perform this process in an acid environment. The stomach secretes hydrochloric acid to create this favorable acidic environment.

However, the stomach does not and cannot supply all the enzymes required for digesting foods. These enzymes can only digest the foods that are already capable of being digested.

Auto-Digestion

Plants, animals and all living matter decay and rot. They turn back into fertilizer for the soil. This process is called auto-digestion. Auto-digestion is normal to the dying processes of all cells. All natural, living or fresh foods automatically digest themselves through the action of their own enzymes.

In order to have value to the body cells and organs, all foods must auto-digest when they are in our stomachs. This means the stomach must first process food nutrients before the body can access and properly use them. Our stomach enzymes and acids work as a team with the enzymes of dying food cells. Without the digestive enzymes of the stomach and pancreas, all foods would decay, putrefy or ferment in our intestines, just as they would decay in a field outside. Instead of nourishing us, the foods we eat would rot and poison us.

Enzymes are destroyed by high heat, chemicals, oxygen, additives, radiation, and microwaves. Overcooked, chemically treated, radiated and microwave foods no longer have the enzymes they need to self-destruct and be digested.

This is also true for foods that are stale and over-processed: all "junk" foods, fast foods, TV dinners, canned food, and most frozen foods. Even before they reach their expiration date, counterfeit, imitation, synthetic and chemically processed foods are lifeless and without value. All these foods are "labeled" as WASTE or JUNK by the stomach for rejection and sent down the chute for elimination at the body's other end.

The stomach also identifies valuable necessary foods. When they come in contact with the stomach enzymes and acid, they undergo a natural change and are transformed into substances that are harmonious with the body's nature. The body can then process, use and thrive on these foods.

It has been shown that white blood cell concentration in the stomach and intestines increases with digestion, since white blood cell enzymes are needed to help with the breakdown and assimilation of food. A person who eats a diet rich in raw food and uses herbs as food and medicine has a plentiful daily supply of enzymes. The enzymes predigest the food in the stomach, sparing the body's white blood cell reserves. This is why a decreased appetite and/or nausea often accompany a disease process.

Digesting cooked or processed foods requires energy at the same time white blood cells are needed elsewhere to fight the disease process. Brain chemistry turns off the hunger center in the brain as needed, so the immune system can be at peak function to fight the disease process.

Stomach Teamwork

Stomach enzymes and hydrochloric acid go to work as a team. The job of this team is mainly to process proteins and minerals.

First, the stomach checks the credentials of every incoming substance. The stomach serves as a loyal health guard. It tags for rejection all substances that come without the supply of enzymes with which Nature always endows them.

Many people might think "the stomach story" ends here, but actually this is just the beginning. Stomach enzymes and hydrochloric acid continue to play a number of extremely important roles in the digestion process.

Hydrochloric acid liquefies and dissolves the food minerals. Only when acted on by this acid are the minerals able to remain in solution, and only in this soluble state can they be absorbed through the intestinal wall. Without hydrochloric acid these minerals would, for the most part, pass through the bowels and be eliminated.

The absorbed minerals dissolve into our body fluids. As part of our blood and body fluids they are carried intact throughout the body and to the cells.

Body cells only recognize those minerals acted upon by the stomach acids and enzymes. When recognized, they are allowed entry and nourish the cells as necessary. However, some minerals manage to successfully by-pass these security measures. By sneaking into the body and circulating throughout, they help balance body fluid needs.

Certain portions of these minerals precipitate the formation of sediment in the tissues. Excess calcium gets deposited into joints. Some calcium forms crystals in the ligaments that surround the joints. These crystals and deposits contribute to creating arthritis.

Calcium may also get deposited in the eyes where it can form cataracts, or in the blood vessel walls where it causes hardening of the arteries; or possibly in the muscles or tendons, creating conditions known as "myositis" or "tendonitis."

Insufficient hydrochloric acid will cause a shortage of calcium. Since calcium is essential to the formation of bones, teeth and nerves for normal functioning of the nervous system and counterbalancing of certain toxic minerals, both hydrochloric acid and calcium shortages can play major roles in conditions such as rheumatoid arthritis, osteoporosis, fluoride poisoning, poor concentration, and low mental abilities.

Without usable calcium, ligaments and joints become weak. They are unable to obtain all the minerals from which they are built.

Calcium is essential for the coagulation of blood during bleeding. In its absence hemorrhaging will occur, activating the production of white blood cells. A calcium deficiency lowers our immunity against blood bacteria and toxins.

Serious shortages of hydrochloric acid affect minerals and favor disease conditions associated with certain minerals, such as:

- **Iron**
    - » Anemia and liver issues. Decreased vitality, mental endurance and strength of will.
- **Iodine**
    - » Lowered thyroid hormones and functions.
- **Magnesium**
    - » Muscle and nerve problems, faulty enzyme systems.
    - » Blocked energy creation, protein utilization.
    - » Lowered protection against infections.
    - » Lowered resistance to stress.
- **Manganese**
    - » Compromised health of bones, ligaments, liver, kidneys.
    - » Lower levels of many enzymes, decrease in mental activities.
- **Zinc**
    - » Pancreas deficiency.
    - » Diabetes.
    - » Liver and skin problems due to deficiencies.
    - » General growth problems.
    - » Poor healing of wounds.
    - » Cholesterol increases.
    - » Fatigue.
- **Potassium**
    - » Loss of endurance.
    - » Sub-performance of adrenals and possibly uncontrollable cell division, leading to cancer.
    - » Decreased healing abilities.

>> Sluggish thyroid.
>> Decreased brain oxygenation.

Undigested protein results in putrefaction, intestinal gas and toxicity.

Infections

Ninety percent of the bacteria that affect our health, and closer to 100% of those that thrive inside our bodies, cannot survive in the presence of a strong acid. This includes the bacteria called "acid fast" (sensitive to acids) bacteria—those which cause tuberculosis. Bacteria and viruses are cell substances; parasites also consist of cells. All of these are digestible, just like ordinary proteins.

Obesity

As soon as you stop a weight reduction program, the weight comes right back on again. You may have gained weight because your body's cells are so de-energized they cannot use their nutrients. Or your weight gain may occur because your digestion has failed to convert your nutrient intake into usable form. Cells become starved. The starvation may have been occurring for years. As soon as food is available, the body eats uncontrollably as it tries to satisfy the starving cells.

The feeling of having had enough at meals comes when the cells are sufficiently saturated and nourished. They may never reach this state without stomach enzymes and hydrochloric acid.

Symptoms of hydrochloric acid and stomach enzyme deficiencies:

* Lack of appetite (possibly the earliest sign).

* Infants who are picky eaters.

* Eating when not hungry.

* Difficulty digesting meats and vegetables.

* Loss of taste for meats and vegetables.

* Fatigue to the point of exhaustion, lethargy.

* Mental fogginess, sluggishness.

* Loss of ambition, enthusiasm, interest in work.

* Irritability, hypersensitivity.

* Burning stomach shortly after meals.

* Nervous stomach; ulcers, duodenal ulcers.

* Fullness, heaviness or discomfort after meals.

* Stomach feels full, even after small meals.

* Stomach cramps and pains shortly after meals.

- Phlegm in the throat; a need to clear the throat.
- A need to blow your nose shortly after meals.
- Belching and burping after meals.
- Lower bowel gas.
- Constipation or constipation alternating with diarrhea.
- Poorly formed stools or noticeable incompletely digested foods in stools.
- Foul odor emanating from the stools.
- Weak joints and ligaments.
- Cold sores (herpes).
- Small hard lumps on the inside of lower lip.
- Hiatus (or diaphragmatic) hernia.

Body changes and signs that indicate low hydrochloric acid:
- Emaciation.
- Pallor.
- Halitosis.
- Smooth surfaced, shiny tongue.

Diseases related to hydrochloric acid and stomach enzyme deficiencies:
- Headaches.
- Anemia.
- Appendicitis.
- Allergies.
- Colitis, Enteritis, Crohn's disease.
- Cancer - 95% of patients with cancer have low HCl. Why is hydrochloric acid not a part of every cancer regime? Why do so few doctors ever prescribe HCl?
- Liver weakness, sluggishness, under-functioning. Foods that are not completely and properly digested cannot nourish the liver. Foods that putrefy or rot, pass through the blood vessels and go directly to the liver where they congest and cause overload.
- "It's all-in-your-head" type illnesses. Since neither deficiency of stomach enzymes nor hydrochloric acid is considered a disease (they are more like a car that has run out of gas), many vague, mild distresses and discomforts are usually disregarded by medics. They are not diseases... "Not-to-worry."

- Acute pain. When hydrochloric acid deficiency and the failure to digest foods become severe, foods start to rot. As they rot they release large amounts of gas that rise and balloon the upper part of the stomach. This presses on the diaphragm and is felt like sharp knife-like pains in the area under the sternum. Sometimes these pains are diagnosed as a heart condition. They can be so severe, even morphine has difficulty controlling them.

- Stomach cramps, nausea, vomiting. The rotting foods turn into "food-poisons." The stomach revolts, causing its muscles to go into contractions and cramps, resulting in severe pains. It does everything it can to eliminate these poisons through nausea and vomiting. It is the stomach's way of protecting the body from holding the poisons inside, i.e., from being poisoned.

- Intestinal or gut cramps. All of the rotting food may not be released from vomit. Whatever passes through the intestines causes similar cramps of the lower intestines.

The positive and encouraging part of the above list is that all of these same symptoms and conditions can be greatly alleviated and even cured by taking hydrochloric acid.

Causes of low levels of stomach enzymes & hydrochloric acid:

- Heredity. About 10% of children are born hydrochloric acid deficient.

- Tension. It affects all areas of the body, even though it is not always felt. Tense nerves that travel to the stomach interfere with and decrease blood circulation.

- Underactive ovaries. Any lack of ovarian hormones contributes to a faulty utilization of proteins and calcium. These keep the nervous systems in balance and free of tension and overactivity. A tense nervous system tightens blood vessels and causes them to contract. This hinders blood flow.

- Insufficient blood circulation, i.e., insufficient nourishment of the stomach tissues and cells and an underproduction of stomach enzymes and acids.

- Overactive adrenals, thyroid, and or pituitary; each of these is a body and nerve activator. They can whip to excess the nerves of the stomach, decreasing the flow of blood and life energies, fatiguing the stomach and decreasing its enzyme production.

- Attitudes and/or lifestyle that create stress and hypertension (anxiety, fears, and worries).

- Insufficient sleep. The stomach can become as tired as the entire body if sleep doesn't replenish the body's energy supply.

- Overwork, burn-out, exhaustion. When our bodies are exhausted our stomachs are just as exhausted.

- Serious deficiencies of minerals and vitamins B-6 and B-2. These affect the stomach and its nerves.

- Irritation of nerves that act on and control the stomach and its functions.

- Displacement of the sixth backbone or neighboring vertebrae, and/or curvatures of the spine in that area. These conditions can compress or irritate nerves going to the stomach.

- Degenerative diseases. About 95% of cancer victims already suffer from a lack of hydrochloric acid. Failure to properly digest foods and the putrefaction of foods that have not been properly digested, contribute considerably to the amount of toxins in our body, our livers and those that get stored in cancer tumors.

- Cigarettes. Inhaling nicotine is almost like gently applying a tourniquet to the circulation of every part of the body—mostly to the stomach.

- Alcohol. It intoxicates and paralyzes nerves and slows down the stimulation of digestive enzyme secretion.

- Moods, emotions and nerves. All of these mental and emotional states can markedly affect the stomach; e.g., "I am fed up," "I can't stomach this or him/her," or, "Don't ask me to swallow that."

It's hard to believe that the inadequate secretion of something as simple as stomach enzymes and acids can have such far-reaching effects on the entire body. Hardly a single part or function of the body is not somehow affected by a deficiency that is so subtle it is often difficult to identify.

How can it be that almost the entire body can be affected by these deficiencies and yet we may not feel sick? Rarely, or at least not until the body wears out with age, do the secretions of enzymes and hydrochloric acid become so low that we experience serious body damage or other symptoms.

This is a sleeper disease, the kind that can be deceptive for years. Then it can "stab us in the back."

Most people may lack only ten or thirty percent of the enzymes and acids they need. This deficiency often goes undetected. One can go for many years, even for most of a lifetime, without being aware of this as a problem. However, with each year of aging, the secretion decreases by approximately one percent. By age 50 or 60, almost everyone is lacking sufficient amounts of both. The body will usually signal these deficiencies.

When determining a deficiency in HCL, avoid:
- Foods that require a large amount of stomach secretions. The worst is milk.

- Excesses of stresses, anxiety, worry, anger, fear, anything that causes tension.
- Overwork, fatigue, exhaustion, non-stop activities with little time for relaxation.
- The use of Tums, Maalox, Mylanta and all antacids. These are the worst products to take when stomach hydrochloric acid is low. They can give you a false sense of wellness by relieving stomach discomforts, at the expense of lowering the cell energies and the electrical energy they produce. Antacids also accelerate aging.

Stomach Ulcers

Ulcers are usually thought to be the result of excess acids. Actually this is a misunderstanding. Stomach ulcers result from too much acid stagnating in the stomach at a time when no more food is present.

Normally, foods dilute the acid and prevent burning, but when food is absent the acid makes direct contact with the skin lining of the stomach and burns it. The stomach is not secreting too much acid. It is secreting beyond its normal time limit, but it is doing this for a reason. Nature makes no mistakes, nor does your stomach. It produces acid not only for digestion, but also for body and cellular needs.

As stated previously, each cell is like a battery (a dry cell) with positive and negative poles. These are acted on by an acid in order to create electricity, which is one of the body's essential energies. The stomach is the source of this acid. When overworked, over-stressed or exhausted, the cells send signals to the brain, demanding that it order the stomach to produce more acid.

With age or after years of answering to these overproduction demands, the stomach becomes tired. Acid production slows down. It cannot produce the full amounts of required acid during meal times, so it merely continues as long as it can or as long as needed, viz., until the body and its cellular needs are satisfied.

A simple proof of this is experienced by taking acid tablets at a time when acids are responsible for acid reflux or burning. A person experiences the same type of relief, whether taking acid or antacid tablets—with one major difference: acid tablets deliver a return to well-being that antacids cannot and will not provide.

Chapter 14

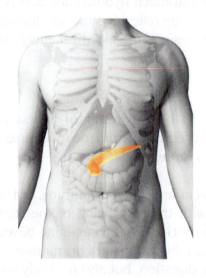

The Pancreas

The pancreas is our biochemical microprocessor.

To most of us and sometimes even to doctors, the pancreas is an organ that is taken for granted. We don't pay much attention to it, nor do we really appreciate it. It works quietly and rarely complains.

We give our pancreas credit for only a minor role in our living and healing, rating it secondary in importance. We know that it helps digest foods, but because we digest our meals unconsciously and seemingly with no effort, we tend to take digestion for granted.

We know the pancreas keeps us from getting diabetes. These are nice and practical services, but we don't think of it as doing anything more.

We overload it, punish it and insult it for years, yet in return, it seems to treat us only with kindness. The vague digestive discomforts and complaints that we experience on occasion are blamed on our stomach. We don't often think of blaming our pancreas. Only when seriously ill do we sometimes become aware of it.

However, we must not be fooled. Overuse or abuse our pancreas, and it will deliver a slow, steady and inevitable decline of our well-being. Illnesses can follow. Constant dietary excesses and deficiencies, stresses and abuses exhaust our pancreases and lead to mild health problems.

The next step can be serious diseases such as:

- Stomach and digestion problems, anorexia.

- Diabetes.

- Celiac disease.

- Hypoglycemia.

- Body toxicities.

- Liver and/or gall bladder conditions.

- Kidney and/or prostate diseases.

- Intestinal conditions: constipation, diarrhea, intestinal gas.

- Colon ailments: colitis, Crohn's disease.

- Diseases of ligaments or bones: arthritis.

- Extreme fatigue and burn-out.

- Headaches.

- Skin diseases: eczema, psoriasis, and others.

- Weight problems: obesity, or progressive losses.

- Mood and emotional swings (sugar-blues).

- High cholesterol.

- Fatty deposits on blood vessel walls, arteriosclerosis, strokes.

- Tumors, Cancer and AIDS.

Every organ of our body is a miracle of marvels and the pancreas is no exception. Much wonderful and "miraculous" living begins in this small, unassuming, quiet, low profile, friendly gland. It protects us against the 18 health problems we've just listed. Without a pancreas our bodies would obtain no nourishment from the foods we ingest and we could not survive.

The almost miraculous role of the pancreas is its ability to produce and secrete large quantities of powerful enzymes that are therapeutic agents as well as food digesters. The pancreas produces and injects insulin into our blood. It is the vigilant curator of our body biochemistry.

How does the pancreas work?

As discussed in Chapter 9, the huge biochemical army of enzymes performs every function involved in living, thinking, feeling, digesting, re-energizing, protecting, healing, restoring, rebuilding, and normalizing cells. Enzymes are responsible for breaking down and eliminating wastes and toxins along with any dying, damaged or foreign cells, tissues or substances.

Pancreatic Enzymes

Before the body's cells and organs can use any food, it must be broken down into biochemical forms or molecule-size building blocks. Pancreatic enzymes perform that pre-absorption process. *No nutrients enter our tissues and cells unless they undergo the impact of pancreatic enzymes.*

Pancreatic enzymes are micro-processors of all foods, both normal and abnormal. The pancreas secretes five main types of enzymes that break down and digest fats, oils, proteins and sugars.

These enzymes are:

- **Trypsin, proteases** - enzymes that split proteins into amino acids.

- **Lipases** - enzymes that change fats into free and readily usable fatty acids and glycerol; these also help to emulsify oils and oil soluble vitamins for cell use.

- **Amylases** - enzymes that split starchy and carbohydrate molecules into absorbable and utilizable sugar molecules.

- **Ribonuclease** - An enzyme that acts on the ribonucleic acid of the chromosomes.

- **Insulin** - transports sugar through the cell membranes and makes it act as fuel for cells.

Pancreatic enzymes work in collaboration with the salivary gland and stomach enzymes. All foods, regardless of their type, are completely digested by the various enzymes of the saliva glands, stomach and pancreas. They complete their tasks within minutes.

The production of enzymes in and by these glands is triggered by pleasurable anticipations of eating and by sensations of seeing and tasting food. The saliva and the stomach enzymes together with hydrochloric acid secreted by the stomach start the breakdown of food molecules and prepare them for their final processing. The presence of hydrochloric acid as it passes into the first portion of the intestines sets into motion the production of pancreatic enzymes.

Enzymes secreted by the pancreas pulverize the various proteins, fats, oils and sugars into specially formatted molecules. All digestion of foods is finalized by the pancreas.

Within a period of a single day the pancreas can produce more than a quart of juices.

All foods must be thoroughly digested. Digesting means reducing foods to sizes and forms that can be absorbed through the intestinal walls and utilized by body cells. If they are not in this molecular form when they pass through the intestines, they will be unable to pass through the gut wall and into the body. They will stagnate in the colon where they will rot, putrefy or ferment.

Inadequate protein type foods rot or putrefy. Sugar foods ferment. The rotting and putrefying of foods creates highly toxic gases. The gases of rotting putrefying protein foods give off a foul odor when they pass out of the body through the rectum. They smell like sulfur (hydrogen sulphide). Gases formed from sugar fermentation have no odor.

Activation of Digestive Enzymes

The entry of foods into the stomach prompts the cells of the stomach wall to secrete hydrochloric acid. This acid is essential to create an acidic environment without which the enzymes cannot start the disintegration of foods by splitting their bonds and breaking them down. All proteins, grains, seeds, sugars and fats are acids.

Only vegetables and herbs are alkaline. The hydrochloric acid of the stomach also changes these into acids.

This hydrochloric acid together with all the acid of the partially digested foods with which it is mixed, flow out of the stomach into the first portion of the duodenum, or first section of the small intestine.

The hydrochloric acid then contacts the cells that make up the duodenal wall. It activates them to secrete and pour into the duodenum a special hormone called "secretin." This hormone passes into the blood and is shunted directly to the pancreas.

Once in the pancreas, the secretin notifies the pancreas that food is on its way and this food will require the digestive actions of the pancreatic enzymes. The secretin activates the production of these enzymes.

The pancreas, now in full production, dumps its enzymes through a special duct which joins with the bile duct from the liver. Through this duct the bile, manufactured by the liver, also empties into the intestines. Together with the pancreatic enzymes, bile mixes with the food.

Bile is a fat emulsifier. For the lipase enzymes of the pancreas to break down and digest fats, the fats must first be emulsified. Emulsification is the fragmenting of fats into minute droplets so the fat handling enzymes can make contact with every molecule of fat—not just the surface portions of the fat foods.

The final stages of food processing start to take place as the pancreatic enzymes—the proteases, amylases and lipases—now exert their actions on the foods entering the intestines. However, pancreatic enzyme activity is possible only when the intestinal environment is alkaline. Bile is also an alkalizer.

Bile combines with alkaline secretions produced by the intestinal wall. By reacting chemically with the acid substances, the bile and alkalines of the intestines change the bulk of the acid meal into alkaline substances.

The action of enzymes on foods

All foods are made up of cells, or in the case of juices, extracts of cells. All cells are made up of proteins and minerals. They also contain molecules of starches and sugars. Cells use these as fuel in order to function. Every cell substance requires special enzymes to pulverize them into micro sizes small enough to pass through the intestinal walls and into forms that the body fluids and cells need and can use.

Digestive enzymes fragment all cells and their components, regardless of the nature of the original food of which they are a part. They destroy all cells whose natures differ in any way or form from the exact individual nature or biochemistry of the cells that constitute our body. They can digest/disintegrate only abnormal cells—cells that are sick, dying, or foreign to the body's chemical identity. These cells have chemical compositions that are different from those of our body.

These enzymes do not and cannot digest or affect any of the normal cells that form the linings of our intestines or the structures of our bodies—at least not until the cells have reached the end of their life span or have become denatured or abnormal.

The chemical make-up of all food cells is different from and foreign to our body. They are all vulnerable to being digested.

Billions of our body's cells wear out and die daily. When this occurs, they become abnormal and foreign to our bodies and are also prey to the actions of digestive enzymes.

These cells require the same types of digestive enzymes that are responsible for the breakdown of food cells.

Digestive enzymes are not destroyed when reacting with cells or other substances. Only gradually do they wear down and become depleted. Nor do these enzymes disappear into thin air or stop existing. Once the digestion of foods is complete, they mix in with the foods and pass together through the intestinal wall where they are transported by our bloodstream into every corner of the body, attacking and digesting every abnormal, denatured, devitalized substance and cell.

This includes sick, dying and damaged cells, and all foreign and undesirable organic substances—everything that is foreign to our body, even bacteria and viruses. The enzymes clear and cleanse the organs and tissues of all the old abnormal cells, cell debris and wastes caused by anything that kills cells, whether they are bruises, injuries, poisons, infections, pus caused by infections, blood clots, stagnating blood, and/or emboli. This also includes cancer cells.

The composition of cancer cells has been damaged and denatured by the poisons, toxins and pollutants that have stagnated too long in certain areas or tissues of our bodies, especially where blood circulation is poor. When these substances are toxic enough, they destroy the particles of chromosomes (oncogenes) that control cell growth, i.e., their process of multiplying and dividing. Anarchy takes over and the cells become tumors.

The pancreas provides favorable conditions for even small quantities of perfectly digested foods to give us energy and perform the cellular repair and healing functions that our body needs.

Insulin also contributes to healing by making it possible for cells to avail themselves of the energies and life forces provided by the burning of sugars. Insulin can assist in the restoration of health in serious degenerative diseases, even cancer.

Pancreatic enzymes support healing processes

For healing, cells need all their special nutrients to replace those used up daily by ongoing metabolic functions. Similar to replacing worn parts of an engine with new ones or adding more wood to a fire to keep it burning, pancreatic enzymes create the new parts and extra fuel.

Healing is accomplished when sick, depleted and/or dying cells are replaced with well nourished, healthy, toxin-free cells. It is estimated that replacing all old cells with new healthy ones can take up to two years. For this reason most healing programs should be followed for up to two years.

By detoxifying the tissues and cleansing them of their wastes and cell debris, the pancreatic enzymes create a clean and healthy environment in which rapid and complete healing becomes possible.

Pancreatic proteases, the protein digesting enzymes, break down, detoxify and eliminate all the microbes that cause infections. Almost all bacteria in our bodies are highly sensitive to acids. They cannot survive in the presence of strong acids. The hydrochloric acid of the stomach plays a major role in protection against and destruction of pathogenic bacteria.

Enzymes protect against allergies

Allergies are the unpleasant reactions we experience as a result of the battle between our enzymes and the enemies of our body that are attempting to destroy our well-being.

They are a demonstration of our system at work, defending itself against antibodies and foreign substances that have invaded our bodies. Most of these allergens are protein-like substances. Therefore, like regular proteins they are digestible by proteases. Allergies that persist over years usually indicate that we are not producing adequate quantities of pancreatic enzymes.

Enzymes are weight correctors

Pancreatic enzymes play a significant role in correcting underweight and overweight conditions.

Underweight and loss of weight are more related to the body's inability to absorb and utilize food than to any other factor. This is usually the result of a poor diet or lack of pancreatic enzymes. When the problem is obesity, the body's innate wisdom knows how to rid itself of fatty tissue and stored wastes. Lipase enzymes together with the bile of the liver, dissolve and digest fats and fatty tissue. Fats are absorbed by and carried out of the body by the bile, lymph and blood. Obesity is a slave to pancreatic efficiency.

Enzymes protect against abnormal cholesterol

Abnormal cholesterols are usually a result of a diet that has excessive amounts of hydrogenated oils, rancid fats and fried foods. These abnormal substances are not easily transformed by digestion into harmless usable food and can be difficult for the body to eliminate.

The fat digesting enzymes of the pancreas play a major role in protecting the blood and artery walls from accumulating these abnormal cholesterol excesses.

A body lacking pancreatic enzymes causes an increase of abnormally high cholesterol levels in the blood.

Enzymes protect against diabetes

An overabundance of sugars in the diet, especially highly refined, processed sugars, enter into the blood in a matter of minutes. Some sugars are used up as they become part of the blood. What is not used causes a rapid rise in blood sugar levels—sometimes to uncontrolled, excessively high levels.

In their natural state, sugars that are whole and that are bound to protein molecules take a longer time to filter through from the intestines and enter the blood. This helps moderate the level of sugar excesses in the blood.

Our body wisdom does not tolerate imbalances and excesses. Blood sugar excesses immediately set into action a counterbalancing mechanism. Insulin is the agent that controls and balances blood sugars. Sugar in our blood triggers the pancreas to produce insulin and release it into the blood. The greater the amounts of sugar, the greater the insulin production that pours into the blood.

Insulin manipulates and controls the cells' use of sugar throughout our bodies. It accompanies sugars as they travel to our cells via the blood. It acts on cell membranes, opening up pore-like passageways in the membranes through which sugar enters the cells. The cells need and use or burn the generous amounts of sugar. However, unless insulin is present, cells cannot receive the sugar that is waiting to be used.

Daily ingestion of excess sugars continued over a period of many years can overwork the insulin producing abilities of the pancreas cells. Eventually and inevitably they become exhausted and depleted. As the pancreas fails to produce the amounts of insulin used by cells to obtain the sugars they need, the sugars are not used up. They start to accumulate and high blood sugar levels result. This condition is known as diabetes.

Blood sugar excesses create another problem as long as the pancreas can produce almost unlimited amounts of insulin. To counterbalance the excesses, our body wisdom immediately secretes equal molecules of insulin for every molecule of sugar. Extra insulin causes the cells to quickly grab large amounts of it from the blood. Sugar levels drop quickly.

The blood is left with levels of insulin that are in excess of' the amounts of sugar. Insulin is more stable. Manipulating cell absorption of sugars does not destroy insulin. It gets used up slowly. Its activity continues for up to 48 hours. At that point the insulin excesses need balancing. Otherwise they will continue to force the cells to absorb sugar. Body reserves will drop and rapidly become drained. Blood sugar levels will continue to drop. When too low, the resulting condition is hyperglycemia.

Diseases resulting from pancreatic enzyme deficiencies

Lack of pancreatic enzymes compromises the digestion process and eventually a health challenge will ensue.

Some of the diseases initiated by the shortage of pancreatic enzymes are:

- **Celiac disease:** A condition resulting from a severe deficiency of most or all the pancreatic enzymes. Foods that are either poorly or totally undigested and their resulting putrefactions wreak havoc on the cells that make up the lining of the small intestines. The integrity of this lining is essential as a barrier to the absorption of unwanted food and toxic substances.

- **Psoriasis:** Faulty digestion and an abused intestinal lining is a condition present in all psoriasis patients. Like all skin diseases, psoriasis is closely related to severe and long term excesses of abnormal, undigested minerals and proteins as well as severe deficiencies of quality oils and the necessary enzymes needed to properly utilize and eliminate them. Toxic substances accumulate, stagnate and build up in the skin. Eventually they cause skin cells to die in excess numbers. Dead/dying cells appear as scaly red patches of skin.

Arch-Enemies of the Pancreas

- **Stresses, Distresses and Negative Emotions:** All abuses and excesses force the body to dip into its reserves. They steal enzymes from whatever organ or tissue is available, resulting in a depletion of our body's reserves of life forces and energies. As our enzyme reserves decrease, they must be replenished or health problems will eventually follow.

Tension-causing emotions (anger, fear, worry, anxiety etc.) overstimulate the nerves. This causes blood vessels to tighten and contract. Blood circulation is decreased, depriving the pancreas of the nutrients and oxygen it requires.

All organs must have constant and complete supplies of each of their specific nutrients. Any element that is seriously deficient compromises the organ requiring that element. The pancreas has a special need, mainly for chromium, zinc, the complex of B vitamins, specific proteins and many trace minerals.

- **Gall Stones:** If a stone blocks the flow of pancreatic enzymes into the intestines, the enzymes will stagnate in their own outlet ducts. The bile will back up into the pancreas canals. This will cause harm to the pancreas.

- **Pancreatitus:** Stagnating pancreatic enzymes attack and even start to digest the blood and nutrient starved cells of the pancreas. This can cause nausea, vomiting and pain that may last for several days.

Chapter 15

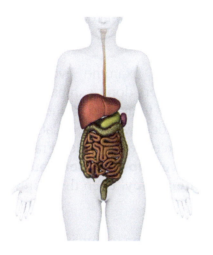

The Liver

The liver is the laboratory of living. It is the ultimate control
center of all diseases and thus is considered the greatest of all living organs.

Health is created, balanced, maintained and protected by the liver.

Whenever illness occurs and persists for any length of time, it should be obvious that some of your body's abilities to protect itself from disease as well as some its healing powers are not performing as they could and should. Your body needs help.

In the course of searching for a way to restore well-being to an ailing body, logic tells us it would be wise to explore the healing mechanism of the body. What organs, biochemical systems and healing agents does our body use to bring about healing? What can be done to mobilize its healing processes in order to help it return to peak condition?

Most doctors and therapists treat the body's obvious needs and symptoms but do not give importance to its key organ of healing. Even holistic oriented doctors that strive to treat the whole person often treat only those negative factors that manifest as disease. They may correct deficiencies, alleviate toxicities, give counsel to the mind, emotions and lifestyle, yet still pay insufficient attention to and provide inadequate support for the healing organ that has to do all the work. Although health stores sell vitamins and minerals, they have few liver remedies. If livers don't scream for help, they don't receive it.

Medical doctors don't generally examine livers. They treat diseases. Liver inadequacies are not diseases. Livers don't exhibit severe symptoms except when severely ill. However, in today's toxic and artificial environment, almost every person's liver is already overloaded with chemicals, drugs, pollutants, and other substances resulting from our excessive lifestyles. Practically every drug adds more side effects detrimental to our liver. **No conscientious doctor should prescribe any drug except in an emergency.** Even then, only in dire circumstances and for a limited time.

If we gave full respect and consideration to our livers, doctors would be left with only a few remedies they could prescribe... and if doctors stopped prescribing drugs, we would witness the demise of powerful drug companies. The medical, drug, hospital and insurance industries won't let this happen.

All doctors and lay persons should be knowledgeable about the liver and liver remedies, yet one can find few books written about the liver. Although scientists have collected massive amounts of information about body cells and biochemistry that includes ongoing studies of the liver and its enzymes, for some reason it is not readily available.

For centuries, herbs for the liver, folklore remedies, homeopathic remedies and liver acupuncture points have been known and used effectively in many parts of the world. Too often, however, they are employed only when obvious signs of liver disease exist. The time we generally treat livers is during periods of abuse, overload and waning health. It doesn't make sense to wait until a disease takes control of your body before giving your liver the care and attention it deserves and needs.

The marvels of our livers

Our livers must be healthy in order for us to survive. Inside this organ the forces of health endlessly battle for supremacy against negative and destructive forces: toxins, wastes, body overloads, excesses, lifestyle abuses and the many abnormalities of our "civilized" living.

Of all the organs in our bodies, the liver is the scapegoat. It gets the brunt of our insults, injuries, stress and hazards.

The most important service we can provide for health protection and disease prevention is an abundance of tender loving care for our livers. When damaged or diseased, our liver has unique abilities to regenerate itself many times over.

The liver is the largest, hardiest and most versatile organ

In the entire body, the liver performs the largest number of functions. It is the hardiest and most versatile of our body organs, possessing almost infinite abilities, functions and levels of stamina. Some of these include powers to heal, normalize and balance all body abnormalities and diseases.

Livers create and store enzymes

As mentioned previously, enzymes are the agents of every function of every organ in the body. Information and research data about enzymes could fill a library. However, little is written about enzymes in regard to therapeutic treatment not only because of their complexity but also because they cannot be manufactured by chemical companies.

Our livers manufacture thousands of different types of enzymes. Some of these enzymes transform the nutrients from the intestines into every biochemical substance the body needs. Use of enzymes for therapeutic treatment is so powerful and effective they could readily replace most drug treatments and put drug companies out of business.

Other enzymes detoxify and render harmless all the wastes and debris of dying cells, worn-out tissues and chemical refuse as well as fumes and garbage generated by all the organs of the body. Enzymes also combine minerals and carbohydrates with toxic substances, rendering them non-toxic so they can be dumped into the intestines and eliminated.

Detoxifying enzymes counteract many of the hazards of our food, water and air pollutants and some of the chemicals, drugs and hazards of our environment. Although extremely powerful, they are not strong enough to overcome all the medical drugs, pollutants, pesticides, radiations and other toxic hazards of modern industry and chemistry.

Enzymes must always be part of all foods and also a part of every supplement. **No food or supplement has healing and normalizing abilities except when functioning in combination with its specific enzymes.**

Our livers create vigor, vitality, and energy

All the cells of our body derive their nutrients and fuel from life-giving nutrients processed by our livers. Thousands of liver enzymes split molecules from food in a manner that is similar to a mini-nuclear explosion. The fission of molecules is a powerful source of our life and life forces.

Liver enzymes transform carbohydrates into glycogen, which is then absorbed and stored by the liver cells. Whenever the body's energy supplies become depleted or when it needs larger amounts for additional activities and stresses, adrenaline, the hormone produced by the adrenal gland, releases this glycogen back into the body. The liver remolds these molecules into readily available sugars that produce energy.

These molecules process starch, sugar, carbohydrates oils and fats. The sugar-fruit-starch meals provide fuel and energy that last only for a short time, however—maybe up to an hour. Liver and body enzymes must be in constant supply because even a few hours of starvation lower liver vitality and function.

For longer lasting durable sources of energies our livers slowly burn and use (metabolize) proteins and oils, thus maintaining a steady flow of energy into the bloodstream. This stabilizes our fuel and energy requirements until the next meal. Without these reserves, starvation and liver devitalization would occur. Serious liver damage can result from this deficiency.

Livers create muscle fuel and energy

Muscles depend on livers for their strength and efficiency. All the fuel foods used by muscles are funneled into the muscles by blood that has been processed and purified by the liver. The liver salvages toxic waste products (lactic acid) from excess muscle activities and changes these back to glycogen.

After the stomach and pancreatic enzymes digest our food, these nutrients pass through the intestinal walls where blood vessels transport them to the liver. Liver enzymes transform them into cell building blocks and materials.

Once processed, the nutrient-molecules are fed back into the blood and carried to every cell and body part where they are used for healing, restoring, repairing and maintaining body integrity and function.

Livers are nutrient "warehouses"

Our livers store oils, sugars, enzymes, cholesterol and thousands of biochemicals. They store vitamins, mainly the A, B, B-12, D, and K groups, and regulate and control the levels of vitamins and other substances in our blood. The liver also stores mineral reserves—mainly iron, zinc, copper, manganese and phosphorus. Our livers provide those vitamins and minerals essential to the creation of blood in our bone marrow.

Proteins and amino acids are also stored by the liver. Proteins must be in molecular food forms that can be transformed into body and liver cells. Only natural unprocessed proteins can be used, stored, or transformed into body and liver cells. The protein cannot be overcooked or chemically treated, hydrolyzed (decomposed by reaction with water), liquefied, or broken into isolated amino acids.

Excess protein concentrations can overload and unbalance the liver. When your liver is troubled, it is best to avoid low quality/high concentrate protein foods or supplements for at least a couple of months.

The liver creates albumin from amino acids. Albumin regulates the body's salt and water balance, an important function, since salt and water imbalance is serious enough to be life-threatening.

Master organ of immunity & resistance

The liver is the organ of body immunity and resistance to disease. It heals, normalizes and controls body biochemicals, stabilizes the body's physical, mental and emotional balance, detoxifies and eliminates toxins.

As the cell builder, healer, master biochemical balancer, stabilizer of substances and nutrients that create inner balance, our livers are also our greatest defense weapons against disease. With a perfectly functioning liver no one would be a slave to any disease. Healing would occur rapidly. Serious health breakdowns or degenerative diseases, including cancer, AIDS, ulcers, multiple sclerosis, arthritis, heart disease, mental and emotional disturbances, kidney, lung, skin or other diseases, would be non-existent. Our livers protect our cells and keep them free from the damages caused by chemicals and pollutants. In our polluted world this is a full-time job.

Master body detoxifiers

Our livers rid our bodies of dangerous excesses of medicines and drugs, body wastes and pollutants, and all health hazards. They are our shock troops, our front line defenders against all abnormalities, chemicals, toxins and poisons.

Liver enzymes combine with all toxic hazardous substances. They eliminate about 40% of all toxins and break down, neutralize, detoxify, and render harmless all substances unnatural to the body, i.e., body poisons, wastes, toxins created by excesses, stresses, fatigue, or products of dying cells.

Possibly the body's most effective detoxifying substance is glucuronic acid, synthesized in the liver with the aid of vitamin C, from glycogen, sugar and lactic acid.

When toxic overloads surpass the liver's capacity to handle them, the liver sends some of these poisons to other organs of detoxification and elimination. The kidneys are the first organs to receive toxic overloads. First, however, the liver must transform these toxins into urea for secretion. Otherwise, our kidneys couldn't dispose of this nitrogen waste.

As cells disintegrate and fragment, they release their histamine, a toxic substance, into their surrounding fluids. Histamine is a chemical irritant that activates and triggers the growth and division of nearby cells. This enables each dying cell to be replaced by a new live and healthy one. Histamine also influences the multiplication and growth of cells in cancer, as these grow into and become tumors.

The liver creates a natural (non-drug) anti-histamine to neutralize body toxins and the histamine secreted by dying cells. The kidneys could not dispose of the high amounts of ammonia, a normal by-product of food and cell degradation as well as faulty protein digestion, without the liver's intervention. The liver converts the ammonia into urea.

Liver biochemicals combat viruses and bacteria poisons, and flush them out of the body.

The liver also manufactures blood clotting/bleeding stoppage substances, such as vitamin K. When hemorrhaging we could bleed to death if it weren't for these control factors created by our livers. The anti-coagulating substance manufactured by the liver is called "heparin." This substance prevents the formation of clots. Without vitamin K or heparin, the formation of clots would block arteries and cause a fatal heart attack or a stroke.

The liver neutralizes and balances sex hormones and sexuality and de-activates excess hormones. It creates, protects and stabilizes our minds and nerves and maintains normalcy for mental abilities and agilities. The sharpness of our brain depends on receiving all the nutrients in blood that has been detoxified by the liver.

Since every drop of blood must pass through the liver, this organ also plays a major role in the control of high blood pressure. Our blood circulation depends on the liver's vigorous handling of all foods and poisons from the blood. Foods that are not properly metabolized and poisons that are not promptly eliminated congest in the liver, causing it to swell up like a sponge. This back-up causes pressure on blood flow, which in turn places stress on the heart.

Organ of elimination
All nutrients and substances that the liver doesn't want or that cannot be used by the body are broken down and/or rendered innocuous by liver enzymes. At the same time it performs this function, the liver manufactures bile that is used as a solvent for absorbing liver poisons. The bile then carries these poisons to the bile ducts and into the intestines where they are eliminated from the body.

Bile
Bile is one of the body's most important agents of digestion, detoxification and elimination. It is a major stimulant of normal bowel movements. The bile and bile toxins irritate the intestinal walls and activate contractions of the intestinal muscles, which in turn force the body to excrete fecal matter.

Poisons cannot be allowed to stagnate in the intestines. If they are not flushed out regularly they will pass through the intestinal wall and the body reabsorbs them. These toxins enter the blood; the blood vessels deliver the impure blood to the liver. What is not flushed out affects the entire body, including the liver.

Problems of elimination result from a sluggish, tired, under-functioning liver. Whenever livers become sluggish, they do not manufacture enough bile. Without adequate bile, elimination of liver and colon wastes and toxins slows down. The vicious circle begins. The bile stagnates, increasing its viscosity or denseness. Bile that is too heavy, like molasses, flows less readily. Transport of toxins and wastes to the intestines is reduced. Stagnating toxins start to build up.

Bile functions:
- The bile in our intestines emulsifies the oils and fats of the ingested foods, including the oil soluble vitamins. Without this emulsification these essential nutrients would not be absorbed.

- Bile dissolves the fatty substances that are stored in fatty tissues. It assists in transporting them to the liver for processing, and then to the intestines for elimination. This procedure can play a major role in the control of obesity.

- Bile absorbs cholesterol and acts as a carrier for bringing this important substance to every tissue of the body via the bloodstream. Bile also rids the body of abnormal toxic cholesterol excesses.

- Normal bile levels decrease excessive appetite and hunger. Its use as a therapy is too frequently disregarded in medicine and by health care practitioners.

The presence of normal, effective amounts of bile is known and recognized by:
- The bowel movement color. It must always be dark brown. When stools are pale brown, yellow or grey, and/or are dry and hard, bile reserves are low.

- Ease of emptying the intestines; absence of forcing.

The thousands of other biochemical transformations that are performed by the liver gives this organ top billing in the human hierarchy as the body's "laboratory," hub or workshop for monitoring and controlling every life function.

Factors that hamper the liver and its functions
Everything that is unnatural, dead and in disharmony with the nature of our bodies can be a hazard to the optimal health and functioning of our livers, and to our health in general.

Our health cannot survive all the current biochemically denatured, polluted conditions of the western civilized world for more than two generations. These destructive forces and abnormalities are so numerous it is not possible to have a healthy, optimally functioning liver.

Pollutants and toxins that our bodies cannot adequately process and release, will stagnate in our livers. They interrupt and hamper the flow of blood and life energies through the liver. Like garbage in a sink they will clog up the liver filters.

Side effects go beyond just affecting the liver. Each organ functions closely with every other organ and energy system of our body. When the life forces of the liver are in plentiful supply and flowing freely, all other organs will be well nourished and functioning as they should. When the liver is no longer able to function normally, almost every other aspect of body-mind performance will be affected.

To retain optimal well-being and healthy livers, we would have to live close to nature... on an idyllic tropical island, free of stress... living true to our individual natures and purposes of living... completely fulfilling our potentials and abilities... picking our food from a tree... and eliminating everything that is negative, artificial, synthetic, chemically treated, devitalized and denatured by the genius of so-called scientific minds. Our lives would have to be free of negatives and all the atrocities we perpetrate on our world, on Mother Nature, and on ourselves.

Everything that hampers digestion—food overloads, stresses and tensions, allergies, etc.—should be eliminated from our bodies and our lifestyle if we are to respect and protect our livers and our lives.

LIVER HAZARDS IN ORDER OF IMPORTANCE

1. Emotional trauma, stresses, negative emotions and attitudes

The organ that relates most closely to our emotional states is the liver. Severe traumatic experiences can do more to undermine and exhaust the abilities of the liver to function normally than months of excessive alcohol indulgence.

By providing all nutrients to the brain and nerves and keeping these areas free of toxins, the liver exerts tremendous influence on all emotions and their control centers.

The emotion that is most closely related to a disturbed liver is anger. Anger is triggered by a congested, slow, sluggish, under-functioning liver. It affects the energies and detoxifying functions of the liver.

Therapies that restore and support the liver play an important role in the treatment of mental states and emotional anguish. Emotions are linked hand in hand with the physiology and energy systems of other organs of the body. Each organ has a special way of functioning that affects the emotions.

2.   Drugs, chemicals, medications, food/water/air pollutants, radiation

All prescribed medications, antibiotics, sedatives, hormones, pleasure drugs, and chemotherapy destroy enzymes and damage the liver. All chemicals force the liver to mobilize enzymes to neutralize their toxic effects, break them down, render them harmless, and eliminate them. Chemicals and drugs destroy liver enzymes and deplete the liver.

When the liver is congested or its function is depressed, except in emergencies all drugs are contraindicated. The use of any drug can block liver restoration as well as all of its functions and healing properties.

Synthetic and the (so-called) "natural" refined, processed vitamins, minerals, and/or amino acids are not foods. They fall into the same category as dead, chemically treated, overheated, refined or processed "foods." They are drugs.

Our bodies can only use substances that are alive or living, in which all their enzymes, minerals, trace minerals and proteins are present. All the elements contained in food substances must be working together in order to successfully nourish, protect and heal our bodies. Every dead junk food or refined processed extract of a food combines with and eventually causes enzyme burn-out. Like drugs, they deplete our reserves of liver and body enzymes.

Radiation is the most destructive of all forces on earth. It devastates and destroys all enzymes and the chromosomes that produce them. Current world atmospheric radiation levels are approximately triple the amount that our bodies can tolerate.

Foods or substances to which the body is allergic act as drugs, toxins, and chemicals. The detrimental effect of foods or substances to which one is allergic is ten times that of the same substances that are readily metabolized by the body.

Stagnant body wastes, cell debris and toxins retained in our bodies by constipation must be eliminated daily in the amount equivalent to the quantity of daily substance intake. For every meal there must be an equal amount of elimination; i.e., one bowel movement. If this does not occur, where is this surplus transported?

3. Lifestyle: excessive habits, failure to exercise and breathe deeply

The diaphragm works with a piston-like action. The down-up expansion and contraction movements of a diaphragm alternately: 1) compress and squeeze toxins and poisons from the liver, and 2) decrease the pressure, thereby creating a vacuum effect that attracts an increase of blood flow to and through the liver.

Lack of sleep, rest, or relaxation deprives the liver of the time it requires to complete its work of breaking down and eliminating poisons and creating the nutrients required by cells. This is only done when the body is at rest and sleeping. Lack of sleep deprives the liver of the time it needs to purify the body and restore all the elements it needs for healing.

In the past, bed rest used to be a standard, universally used therapy. It is still an extremely effective way to restore health.

Sleep should be part of a good liver regime.

4. Dietary excesses, abuses, toxicities, and deficiencies

Anything and everything that is unnatural, chemically treated, excessive and radioactive can be a serious hazard to our livers. Livers cannot remain healthy when burdened with instant, denatured, artificial, canned, processed, radiated, stale, colored, "preserved" junk and dead foods. It cannot transform dead "foodless" foods into molecules needed and utilized by body cells.

Heating foods above 165 degrees Fahrenheit or 70 degrees Centigrade destroys enzymes and about 95% of proteins. The higher the heat the more destruction.

Overeating overloads the liver. The liver is like a sponge, taking in or "sopping up" food excesses. This excess clogs the millions of filters our livers use for purifying blood and causes liver fatigue. Food excesses also require excessive amounts of enzymes to metabolize them. Enzyme reserves can be depleted.

5. Alcohol, soft drinks and synthetic beverages

Note that alcohol is not the only or most important cause of liver ailments. We have ranked it fifth here.

Chemical flavorings, colorings, preservatives, additives, pesticides and chemical fertilizers have a far greater effect on livers than the alcohol itself. There are more chemicals in commercial cheaper wines, beers and liquors than in most foods. All of these force the liver to use up large reserves of their enzymes, especially those of the vitamin B complex groups.

6.   Common diseases arising from liver problems

Anyone affected by ill health that persists for any length of time has lost the protecting, rebuilding and maintaining powers of their liver. This life-sustaining organ is losing its battle against endless abuses, maltreatments and neglects. It is breaking down under constant and extreme overloads.

When livers don't function as they should, we can experience any, or many of the following symptoms:

- **Breakdown of immunity - host resistance**

- **Exhaustion, fatigue, burn-outs**

- **High blood pressure:** All blood returning through the body after being pumped by the heart must pass through the liver. When the liver is congested, this pressure back-up interferes with blood flow. The blood has difficulty moving through the liver. The heart continues to pump blood that pushes against this obstruction, causing a build-up of blood volume and increased pressure against the blood vessel walls. This scenario often causes increase in blood pressure.

- **Thrombosis:** When blood cannot circulate freely through the liver, it stagnates. This can produce clots.

- **Fatty Livers:** Fatty livers are caused by prolonged deficiencies of choline, liver enzymes and vitamins; excesses of fats and chemicals in our diets; overfeeding; body toxins; tobacco; drugs; arsenic; phosphorus; alcohol; and similar pollutants. Poisoning of the liver cells interferes with metabolism.

  In the same way that fat deposits develop when wastes and excesses accumulate beyond the body's enzyme supply and ability to eliminate them, the liver also becomes a storage bin for fats, food excesses, harmful wastes, toxins and poisons that accumulate and stagnate.

  The liver is protected against fat accumulations in its tissues by the action of pancreatic enzymes, and by choline (a B vitamin that emulsifies fats) and inositol.

- **Kidney Diseases:** Excess toxins that the liver is unable to handle overflow into the kidneys, which then releases them.

- **Disturbances of fat metabolism:** Psoriasis, schema, acne, skin rashes and other skin diseases are caused by disturbances of fat metabolism. Fat foods are digested by pancreatic enzymes. Once digested, they are processed by: 1) special oil/enzyme factors of the liver, 2) choline, and 3) the bile.

During World War I in central Europe, there was a severe shortage of oils. Even abnormal toxic oils were unavailable. Diseases such as psoriasis that are manifestations of toxicity by abnormal oils became so rare, medical students had little or no opportunity to see or study a case. When the war ended and fats and oils, both good and bad, were again available, the incidence of psoriasis returned to pre-war levels.

Psoriasis almost disappeared in Japan during the war of 1945-47 when the country experienced widespread food shortages. According to Dr. Ito of Kanazawa University of Japan, an increase of psoriasis cases parallels the increase of pork fat in the Japanese diet.

- **Pneumonias and lung diseases**
- **Cirrhosis of the liver:** Cirrhosis is a state of liver degeneration whereby fat cells replace a great number of the liver cells that died or degenerated from lack of proper nutrition and care, and from the effects of toxins, drug overloads and poisons. When contact with the poisons is too prolonged or they are present in excess quantities, cirrhosis and death can result.

  Cirrhosis is acclaimed by the medical profession as incurable. The fact is, however, *it is incurable only if drugs are used as therapies*. By fulfilling all the liver requirements with health restoring regimes, diets and therapies, it is possible over a period of years for the liver to grow back to normal. This assumes the condition is not too advanced or extreme.

- **Hemorrhoids:** Hemorrhoids are not really a disease. They are a symptom, a red flag the body uses as an S.O.S. or danger signal indicating the liver is overloaded and swollen.

  When the liver is seriously congested, blood circulation is hampered. The pressure back-up extends through the veins down to those in the walls of the rectum. These expand and swell. The blood flows sluggishly. Surrounding tissues become starved for nutrients and oxygen. Whenever this occurs anywhere in the body, our body wisdom sends a message in the form of an itching, to whatever area is affected. The itching makes us want to scratch and the scratching again increases the flow of blood.

  Rectal bleeding occurs when buildup of blood in the rectal veins causes breakage of these veins. Rectal veins are some of the thinnest and weakest in the entire body... a skillful maneuver of body wisdom.

As blood volumes build up with the potential for blood vessel breakage, we do not want the bleeding to happen inside the body. This would be fatal. The blood will flow outside the body.

Hemorrhoids are a life saving protective mechanism. Hemorrhoid veins should not be surgically removed. This also removes valuable warning signals about high blood pressure or liver congestion. Instead of surgery, treat hemorrhoids by decongesting the liver, or by ridding the body of any other obstruction or pressure that is blocking the blood flow. The hindrance could be from pregnancy, tumors, or constipation.

- **Diabetes and livers:** About 80% of patients with fat saturated livers are pre-diabetic. The liver is the storehouse for body sugars. Any additional body needs, stress or stimulation can trigger the liver to dump too much sugar back into the bloodstream. Excess sugars deplete insulin reserves and predispose the body to diabetes.

- **Congestion of the brain and nervous system:** All the blood from the brain has to pass though the liver, which filters and removes the toxins and replaces its nutritional supplies.

  Blood coming from all parts of the body, including the upper body—the brain, nerves, eyes, ears, and sinuses—cannot flow freely through a liver that is already overloaded with metabolic and catabolic products. If the toxins don't get filtered out of the blood, they will stagnate in the brain. Toxins can affect the brain in the same manner as alcohol excesses.

- **Migraines:** As already described, a congested liver means a congested brain. Congestion is blood stagnation. Stagnated blood becomes toxic, like the water of a blocked river turning into a swamp. Poisons or irritants that contact nerve endings in the brain as well as in the body trigger a warning signal of their presence. This signal is felt as pain. Such pains can be in the head or in any part of the body.

CARE FOR YOUR LIVER

Without liver care and support, there would be no health or life. First, it is important to know and understand how to care for the liver and address any potential hazards that could damage it. There's no point in swallowing pills or liver restoring supplements if little or no attention is paid to the causes of liver problems and to all of its requirements. This means careful avoidance of all toxins, body pollutants, chemicals and poisons; and complete elimination of their stagnation.

It is more important to get toxins, wastes, poisons, drugs and chemicals out of the body first, before trying to nourish or rebuild the liver.

Liver care means:

1. Having the same number of daily bowel movements as substantial meals. What goes into the body must come out.
2. Living with positive emotions, attitudes and outlooks.
3. Avoiding all excesses.
4. Providing the liver generously with every nutrient and element required to rebuild all of its cells, thus making it possible for the body to function optimally.

As important to the liver as eating or any therapy are:
(Their importance is in the order given.)

- Detoxifying and eliminating liver hazards

- Positive, attitudes, emotions and morale

- Joyous lifestyle

- Good regular exercise

- Clean unpolluted air

- Living natural foods

Restore and maintain positive attitudes, emotions and outlooks to create a joyous, fulfilling lifestyle. Avoid all lifestyle/ habit excesses. Exercise, exercise, exercise. Breathe deeply and often. Provide every nutrient and element required to restore and rebuild liver cells and their functions.

For optimum liver health, avoid the following foods:

- **All synthetic foods -** T.V. dinners, NutraSweet, Aspartame and artificial sweeteners, cream substitute coffee mixes (every ingredient of Coffee Mate is a chemical or drug).

- **Wheat foods -** White flour and flour products. Man-made strains of wheat contain five times more gluten than Nature's original strains. Gluten makes our blood and body fluids become thick like glue—just as when you mix flour and water. This can create serious circulation problems. Excesses of this kind of wheat can markedly congest and plug up the liver.

- **All commercial boxed, dry, (sweetened) cereals -** Corn Flakes, Total, and all cereals similar to these.

- **All refined foods -** Those from which the natural content of vitamins, minerals, enzymes and/or life forces have either been eliminated by commercial extraction and processing, or destroyed by heat, oxygen, chemicals or radiation.

- **All rich foods -** Sweets, desserts, white sugar, "ice creams," candies, jellies, syrups, "diet foods," cookies, chocolate bars, jams, etc.

- **Sugar excesses -** One can get too much of even the quality sugars, including honey. Use honey only if unpasteurized. Use only up to 2 – 3 Tablespoons daily. The maximum body tolerance of sugars from any source is 4 ounces.

Sugars from high sugar/starch breakfasts absorb rapidly into our blood. This pushes up our blood sugar levels quickly and excessively. The pancreas comes to our defense by secreting large amounts of insulin to balance these sugar levels. This insulin burns up the excess sugars in a very short time. However, it also continues to burn sugars that are supposed to be maintained in reserve in our bodies, livers and blood. This process lasts for up to forty-eight hours. Our blood sugar levels will then drop very low, causing hypoglycemia.

Our liver sugar levels also drop. The liver cannot function without large amounts of sugar. An under-functioning liver is the result. Our brain sugar levels also drop, causing decreased brain abilities. Our brains use as much sugar as the rest of the body.

- **All soft drinks, sodas, synthetic and artificial fruit juices.**

- **All rancid, old, stale, chemically treated, commercial oils** - All grocery store salad dressings, mayonnaises, stale, rancid, hydrogenated oils, margarines, peanut butters, spreads, etc.; all non-vacuum packed wheat germ and its oils.

- **All fried foods** - Don't use fats or oils in combination with high starch, sweet and sugary foods. These adhere to and coat the outer surfaces of foods. This coating makes it impossible for the stomach and pancreatic enzymes to make contact with the food substances to digest them. The undigested foods rot or putrefy in the gut.

- **All high fat foods** - Pork, ham, bacon, lard, Crisco, shortenings, French fries, chips, and fried foods.

- **All preserved foods, food additives, food chemicals, food colorings, flavorings and thickeners** - There is no such thing as a preservative. To preserve is to mummify. The so-called preservatives are "embalming fluids." To mummify is to destroy the life forces and enzymes of foods. The most destructive form of food preservation is radiation. It destroys foods just as it destroys the human body.

- **All (so-called) smoked meats, fishes, foods.**

- **All canned foods, vegetables, fishes and meats** - Canned tuna and salmon, especially.

- **Frozen Foods** - Except for frozen beans/seeds (corn, peas, beans), use only fresh vegetables whenever they are in season.

- **All re-heated, long-stored foods** - The longer a food is stored, the less nutritious and more lifeless it becomes.

- **All microwave or pressure cooked foods, and overcooked foods–** Powerful microwaves physically shatter and thus denature protein molecules so they can no longer be assimilated. Denatured proteins are toxic. They reduce immunity and resistance to disease and contribute to cancer and cellular degeneration.

- **Enzyme-deficient foods and supplements -** This includes vitamins and minerals and isolated amino acids.

- **All processed protein foods -** Baloney, wieners, salami, canned meats, etc. These are also denatured and toxic.

  Like chemicals, foods also undergo chemical reactions. Acid foods react with alkaline foods, causing them to denature each other, thus becoming unusable by the body. Even eating the best of foods can deprive the body of nutrients when this occurs.

Foods to be used in moderation (for optimum liver health):

- **Starches, high gluten foods and breads -** At best, breads are overcooked, highly concentrated starches, so the less the better.

- **Flesh meats -** Preferably, use wild game meats, lean meats, fowl, and chicken (only when and if they are healthy or organic).

- **Citrus fruits and especially their juices -** Taken in excess the citric acid in citrus fruits binds itself to calcium, turning it into insoluble and unusable salts or crystals. These crystals can deposit in our joints and cause pains and arthritis.

- **Large quantities of fruits at any one meal -** Taken as a breakfast, they trigger too much insulin production. This induces a hypoglycemic state for up to 48 hours.

- **Eggs -** One to three eggs a day is acceptable, if they are healthy. Healthy eggs do not increase blood cholesterol levels since they contain lecithin, which burns up cholesterol. To be healthy the eggs must be:
  - » From healthy, range fed chickens.
  - » Fertilized.
  - » Only lightly and slowly cooked, not beyond softness (never fried or hard boiled).

Foods that promote health in the liver:

- **Natural foods -** Living, undercooked, or uncooked (never micro-waved or pressure cooked), chemically free, unadulterated, grown on naturally fertilized (no chemicals or pesticides), completely mineralized soils.

  The liver tolerates only natural live foods and natural liver supplements.

The liver uses larger amounts of the vitamin A and B groups than any of the other vitamin complex groups. Liver functions are most depleted and damaged when deprived of vitamin A and B enzyme groups.

- **High quality protein diets -** The liver cannot subsist or function without a generous supply of quality proteins. These are foods that provide all the amino acids in an excellent balance. They must be in constant supply. Even a few hours of depriving the liver of these amino acids lowers its vitality and functions. A quality protein must be part of every meal. **One quarter of the usual daily food intake should be protein.**

These proteins must always be taken in natural nutrient forms that can be transformed into body and liver cells. Proteins must never be overcooked, chemically treated, hydrolyzed, or isolated into single amino acids.

Flesh meats, soy beans, and millet are forms of high quantity (high concentration), but low quality proteins. High protein concentrations can overload and unbalance the liver. When your liver is troubled, avoid these until it is well.

Proteins restore and sustain the liver; they also satisfy and relieve hungers and cravings for excesses of foods, sweets, alcohol, or cigarettes. All of these are harmful to the liver.

Proteins that contribute most to optimal liver health are:
- **Internal organs from healthy, organically raised animals (liver, sweetbreads, heart, kidney, tongue -** To preserve their food value, prepare them by lightly broiling.
- **Brewer's yeast -** A liver tonic. Protects liver functions.
- **Seeds, grains -** Whole, soaked 48 hours, freshly ground, crushed.
- **Nuts -** In shells, not roasted or salted. Best are almonds, hazel nuts, and walnuts.
- **Deep ocean fish-** Halibut, sole, salmon.
- **Eggs -** only if healthy; range fed, hen fertilized (1 - 2 a day; cook lightly; never hard boil or fry).
- **Juices -** Live food concentrates with their enzymes and vitamins. If you have a juicer, make juices fresh from carrots, apples, beets (roots and leaves), cucumbers, apples, and dandelion leaves (organically grown if possible).

Oil/Enzyme complexes:

Oil deficiencies are more common and detrimental to health than vitamin and mineral deficiencies. Usually only those who have made a study of quality foods and oils get enough oils. Possibly this is because most people have been taught to identify oils with fats and calories. They still freely use salad oils, mayonnaises, margarines and sandwich spreads from the local grocery store.

High quality oil rich foods - The liver functions poorly without substantial amounts of food oils. These foods provide essential oil soluble vitamins and trigger the flushing of the liver and its bile.

The following seeds and their oils (when they are cold pressed) are the most nutritious:

- **Sesame, sunflower, safflower, flax, wheat germ.**
- **Nuts, seeds, grains, cereals.**
- **Peanut or almond butter** if made from freshly shelled, lightly roasted nuts, with a little sea salt and oil added.

Each oil contains more of certain nutrients than others. To get the most benefits, it is best to mix several kinds together.
Our bodies and livers need 2 - 3 Tablespoons daily.

You can buy special oil/enzyme complexes essential to provide therapeutic benefits in diseases caused by toxic oils or from a lack of hormones.

These are:

Gamma Linolenic Acid - This is commonly known as Primrose Oil. It is found in many other forms from other sources and plays an important role as a protective coating for cell membranes and chromosomes. Linolenic Acid reinforces the immune systems.

Choline - A fat dissolver, mobilizer and eliminator. Choline protects the liver against fatty degeneration. It also transforms fat in the liver into lecithin, making it fat soluble and transportable. Taking processed lecithin blocks this process.

Arachidonic Acid - A fatty acid essential to health. These quality oils provide therapeutic benefits in hormone production for skin conditions (psoriasis, eczema, acne, dry scaly skin and dandruff, etc.).

Methionine - The liver needs and uses this amino acid to manufacture choline and lecithin. Choline and lecithin are essential for the metabolism, transportation and mobilization of fats, oils, cholesterol and sterols and for the production of hormones.

Vegetables and fruits – the most beneficial to the liver:
- Salads (hot/cold); a large variety of greens
- Baked potatoes, brown rice
- Carrots, beets, dandelion greens, radishes
- Parsley, celery, rhubarb, artichokes, endive
- Vegetable broths

Use liver in the diet as a liver therapy. Nothing is as perfect for livers as livers. When healing from a serious illness, patients can hardly eat enough liver to make up for years of abuse and liver starvation.

Obtaining quality liver can be a problem. In order to be a health giving food, it would have to come from healthy animals that have been allowed to roam free on the range; choosing foods that their instincts tell them are what they need for their health. These are foods from soils and plants untouched by chemical fertilizers and pesticides.

For people who are too ill to look after themselves, obtaining and preparing their own health restoring foods may be nearly impossible. The best alternative is supplements: liver extracts in a concentrate pill size form. One can find many other wonderful liver foods and herbs, but no plant or food contains every element and nutrient that is in the liver.

Animals of prey instinctively know about the value of livers. When a lion downs a prey, it feasts on the liver first, often leaving the muscle meats and less valuable remains of the quarry to scavengers, birds and rodents. The values of the different nutrients show in the strength of the lion and weakness of the scavengers.

Liver Supplements:
Among thousands of companies that sell vitamins and minerals in America, only a few develop products capable of restoring optimal health and function to livers.

Such concentrates must not be heated and they must not be treated by chemicals, refined or processed. They must retain life forces needed to replace those used up by livers in their fight against all the pollutants of civilization. The liver restoring and healing powers or their enzymes must not have been destroyed or lost through manufacturing processes.

 If liver congestion has been a problem for a long time, it is advisable to take a good quality yucca extract (I recommend "Optimum D-Tox") once or twice a day.

"Optimum D-Tox" is a proprietary concentrated extraction of schidigera yucca that contains numerous plant enzymes, phyto-nutrients and saponins that assist in breaking down and eliminating rancid fats, along with stagnant surpluses of body toxins and wastes; thus reducing stress on the liver.

Lifestyle activities beneficial to the liver:

- **Exercise:** Deep breathing exercises are especially good. Breathe in as deeply as you can and hold for 2 – 3 seconds. Breathe in again, deeper. Hold your breath for as long as you can comfortably do so. Slowly and gradually breathe out.

  This type of breathing exercise causes the diaphragm to press down on the liver and force out blood and toxins. The upward movement of the diaphragm allows for and aids liver expansion and inflow, or greater quantities of blood from the body together with the "new" toxins and wastes that need to be processed by the liver.

  This type of breathing is even more effective if done when trying to touch your toes, either while standing up or sitting down.

- **Sleep**: The liver needs rest and time to perform its functions. It also needs to catch up with the backlog of unutilized or unmetabolized substances. Cutting back on hours of sleep needed to feel energized and refreshed does not give the liver sufficient time to break down and eliminate wastes and toxins accumulated during the previous day's (or month's) activities. Substances not processed during sleep hours will accumulate in the liver.

  Shortened sleeping hours accumulated over months or years cause congestion of the liver. Poisons that stagnate will eventually act on and damage the liver cells. Getting lots of sleep is as important as other therapies for liver restoration.

How long do our livers need special care?

Usually the body requires about one year of therapy for every ten years of illness, health problems and liver abuse. One must be watchful and cautious until full health is restored.

Reactions that may occur during healing:

The more intense and effective a therapy, the greater the chance of experiencing discomfort at some time during the healing process. Some of these discomforts or distresses will be upsetting and cause anxiety. For many centuries we have been conditioned to believe that every unusual and uncomfortable change in the ways our bodies are feeling or functioning is an evil. Therefore, our first impression usually is to assume that the treatment we are taking isn't right for us and is creating harmful side effects.

If you properly understand what healing is all about, you will realize the body has an inborn wisdom. This wisdom means that our bodies make no mistakes. When a liver reacts in an unpleasant way, it is merely reminding you that it is working overly hard and also working overtime. It is tired.

Each time you dump toxins, wastes and poisons back into your blood from body storage areas, you overload your liver. Every effective therapy that you use, forces the healing processes of your liver to work harder. This additional stress may cause your liver to complain or rebel by developing symptoms and distresses.

These symptoms are called healing reactions (sometimes referred to as a healing crisis).

No organ is more easily affected by external influences than the liver. Whenever you are carefully following a regime that is tailored to your healing needs and experience what seems to be a setback or an unpleasant reaction to this program, your body is trying to tell you it needs to rest. It needs time to catch up with its overload of toxic dump. It is working beyond its abilities.

The most effective relief at this time would probably be to halt all the therapies that are increasing the work load on the liver and go on a fast. For a time, eliminate all the foods and supplementation that are making your liver work harder so you can give it a chance to metabolize, detoxify and eliminate excesses that are tiring and upsetting it.

You should experience some relief within a few days. Taking "Optimum D-Tox," as suggested earlier, will accelerate this process.

Allow your body to once again feel good (usually this takes a couple of days) and then resume your healing regime.

Take care of your liver. It cannot be replaced. When your liver goes, you also lose your health, immunity, vitality, emotional and physical well-being—and peace of mind.

Learn to abide by the laws of nature by eliminating anything that is negative, artificial and/or denatured.

There is nothing we will ever do that will improve on what the Creator abundantly provided for us in nature.

The best way to maintain a healthy liver is to subscribe only to those disciplines that keep the whole body in a state of optimal health. Wellness is not the result of your physician…it is the result of your self-care!

Chapter 16

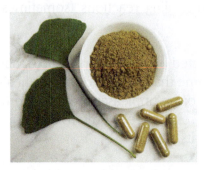

Herbs

Potential therapeutic values of herbs

Since herbs are man's main source of therapeutic enzymes, our first search for a means to conquer degenerative conditions should influence us to learn about these miraculous healing catalysts or agents.

First, it is important to note that herbs must grow in their proper environment in order to have their full healing potential.

Second, although they are foods, usually they are not normally consumed as a part of our daily diet.

For an herb to be scientifically categorized as a legitimate treatment of a specific disease or remedy for any particular patient, the precise quantity and nature of the enzymes of that herb and the specific need of the individual for those enzymes would have to be known. Only those herbs or enzymes which a person lacks or particularly needs could succeed in supporting the normalizing of that individual's biochemical ratios.

Those who continue to adhere only to the philosophy that tumors are evil, i.e., lethal enemies, may persist in believing these wicked predators must be cut away or destroyed. They may continue to believe that the only forces that are powerful enough to kill cancer cells are drugs and radiation. We must, however, realize that poisons strong enough to kill cancer cells also kill healthy cells.

They cannot have understood enzymes. Nor do they realize that you don't have to poison cancer cells. They can be destroyed just as readily and effectively by disintegrating or digesting them through the use and action of enzymes.

Chromosomes and enzymes are destroyed by:

- The action of oxygen. In plants and foods, oxygen creates toxic staleness. In oils, it creates toxic rancidity.

- Excess heat, overcooking and pressure cooking. The higher the temperature above 165 Fahrenheit (75 Centigrade) the greater the enzyme destruction. In fact, whenever the temperature rises above normal body temperature, enzymes begin to be destroyed. Microwaves are powerful vibrations that physically shatter proteins and enzymes.

- Fluorides, including those found in our drinking water, tooth pastes and dental treatments. Fluorides are among the most powerful enzyme destroyers known to chemistry research.

- Radiation, cobalt, Cat scans, X-ray pictures.

- Chemicals, drugs, poisons, carcinogens, chemotherapy, pain killers, sleeping pills, sedatives, pesticides, aerosols, preservatives, prescription drugs, excess accumulations of body toxins, and body wastes. Even mild drugs like aspirins damage enzyme activity and therapy efficiency.

- A substance is a poison only because it reacts with, damages, wears out, depletes, and/or destroys enzymes and proteins.

- The intake of dead, canned, frozen, rancid, irradiated, refined, processed, chemically treated, and synthetic foods—including vitamins, minerals and amino acids that are devoid of their enzymes. The label "From Natural Sources" means only that it originally came from something in nature but bears little or no statement of its present condition.

   For example: petroleum is a natural product, but a synthetic vitamin made from petroleum is not something that a prudent person would want to force upon their body. Refining and processing kills all enzymes.

All minerals in their pure form, e.g., lead, iodine, iron, aluminum, nickel, selenium, germanium, copper, zinc, sodium, potassium, magnesium, manganese, cobalt (as in, vitamin B-12), etc., use up and destroy enzymes.

Metals and minerals can only be effectively used by the body when they exist in their proper form. For example, in chemistry there are two forms of iron: ferric and ferrous. One is used to make steel, the other works far better in the human body. One can take herbs with biologically less functional forms and convert them into far more useful ones for human physiology if properly prepared, so that none of its enzymes are destroyed or missing. These can be used by the body and remain valuable as therapies.

Anything that prevents this biological conversion and damages or destroys chromosomes and enzymes also destroys cell integrity, function, structure, immunity and resistance. It blocks healing and threatens the very life of our bodies.

Effectiveness of herbs as healers

The molecular structure of the cells can be restored if the therapies used provide all the necessary nutrients for the body to correct every cellular need and imbalance.

Because of their ability to detoxify the body, enzymes are major control agents of pain.

Benefits of herbal enhancement of host resistance and immunity should be:

- Improvements of body physiology and healing abilities.
- Increased well-being, vitality, enthusiasm for living and general well-being.
- Correction of body deficiencies.
- Renewal of enzymes, immunity, and resistance reserves.
- Specific strengthening of body organs.
- Pain relief by neutralizing and eliminating toxins and poisons.
- Relief of many or all distresses and symptoms.

Precautions before and during herbal therapy:

- Avoid all drugs, chemicals, chemotherapy, and radiation.
- Avoid even the strong pain killers, sedatives, sleeping pills, preservatives, food additives, contaminants, fluorides, pesticides, industrial waste disposals and other pollutants.
- Avoid using synthetic vitamins and minerals or chelated minerals—even those from health stores.

Many brands of vitamins and minerals are generally refined, treated with chemicals, isolated from their teammate proteins, minerals, trace minerals and oils. They are still labeled "from natural sources" even though they have lost their healing ability.

When following a regime, other modes of treatment should not be used without notifying your doctor (or all of your doctors) and explaining your procedures.

Do not use digestive enzymes within 3 hours before or after taking herbs and herb teas. These can possibly change some trace mineral/protein/enzyme compositions of the herbs.

Amounts of herbs that are advisable

In early stages of a disease when tests indicate that causes of disease are present or that small tumors are starting, a small dose of a specific herb(s) every day or every second day can often be effective. This amount can sometimes be enough to control or slow tumor growth, or gradually decrease its size.

Generally, herbal remedies should be taken twice or more daily. Doses should be progressively increased until the body undergoes a noticeable change.

Changes can be:
- Experiences of improved well-being.
- A change of symptoms.
- A reaction to the remedies—either pleasant or unpleasant.
- Some form of a healing crisis.

After 4 - 5 days, if no response is experienced or if there is no progress or improvement—no reduction in the sizes of the tumors, appearance of other symptoms, or healing responses—increase the amount of the remedy you are taking. Initially prescribed remedies and doses are intended mainly as tests, both of body tolerance and effectiveness.

To prevent recurrence of disease and tumors:
- Communicate with your doctor regarding your observations and experiences. He depends on your information to keep the treatments in balance, conforming with your body needs.
- When symptoms have cleared and tumors have been removed or destroyed but all the abnormalities that caused your condition have not yet been annulled, eliminated and resisted, continue with maintenance doses of your remedies. Stay with this program for several months after all signs of disease have left. The amounts of the specific herbal remedy to be taken should be progressively diminished.

When treatments don't deliver expected results:

Healing has ups and downs. Everyone enjoying excellent health experiences these highs and lows. Even if one is following a therapy that is working, the pattern will be the same. The body will continue to go through cycles—periods of healing followed by periods of detoxifying. The healing periods are experienced as highs and the detoxifying periods as lows.

Consider that it takes energy to run your body and also to heal. If there's not enough energy to do both, the intelligence that runs your body will stop the healing process and you will coast while it builds up its energy reserves. During this time you will not feel as well as a few days before. When the energy reserves are restored, healing will again begin. Therefore, it is vital that you obtain as much rest as possible during these periods.

Whenever one is involved in a therapy that is incapable of creating any "wrongs" and something still feels "wrong" or is sensed as wrong, actually it is the causal factors of the disease leaving the body. They are being dumped from their storage tissues back into the blood and body fluids. During this process they contact nerves or temporally poison tissues and create unpleasant sensations.

If tumors do not show signs of decreasing in size or do not respond to the therapy, chances are, something else is wrong. Your treatment may be a good one for someone else, but not for you. It is not tailored to your body's needs.

To correct this situation:

- It is necessary to eradicate the possibility of a missing problem or imbalance. More discussions with your doctor or more testing and/or investigations may be necessary.

- It may be that a more precise balancing of your regime is needed. One unsolved problem, one untreated causal factor may and often does suffice to block the efficiency of an otherwise very effective treatment. This includes an evaluation of your mental attitude. A person who has resigned themselves to die most certainly will die in spite of proper care.

- Your immunity/resistance/life/healing forces are depleted.

- Knowingly or unknowingly, you are not following your program accurately and consistently.

- A good re-evaluation of the nature and causes of your condition is seriously needed. Not enough has been understood, diagnosed or revealed, or clearly understood about your condition. Causes of your condition are still present and active. Something is blocking your body's healing abilities.

Every therapy and its healing potential are affected by:

- Personal experiences.

- Personal reactions to those experiences.

- Lifetime conditioning and mindsets.

- Personal attitudes and outlooks.

- Willingness and good will. Without a patient's acceptance and cooperation, no therapy can be effective.

Chapter 17

Colds, Coughs, Fevers & Flus

Be kind to yourself... you are all you've got.

Colds, coughs, fevers and flus have several things in common:

- None of these conditions is a true disease. Because they are not diseases there are no "cures."
- Each is a normal reaction of our body's innate wisdom responding to a challenge arising from excess body pollutants.
- Each is a process of dumping or destroying excess body wastes.
- Even though viruses or bacteria are present, they are only part of the pollution process. *They are not the primary cause.*
- They can be effectively cured without drugs or antibiotics.

Exactly what are these conditions?

For generations these four conditions have been classified as "diseases." For centuries people have viewed every physical state of the body that is not comfortable, normal or "perfect" as an evil.

The French word "malady" means "disease." "Mal" means "bad, wrong, evil." However, the evil is in the *cause*, not in *the body's reaction to the cause*.

Currently we are living in the most polluted, toxic and chemically hazardous era this planet has ever experienced. It is not possible to take a breath of air, drink of water or mouthful of food without absorbing hazardous pollutants or chemicals. Daily we absorb chemicals, pesticides, additives, synthetics, denatured foods and pollutants.

Thirty thousand toxic substances have been added to our foods and hundreds more exist in our air and water. Our environment contains over 100,000 harmful substances and chemicals. In our bodies, several billion cells die daily. If not metabolized properly, each of these cells is like a microscopic cadaver that rots and disintegrates in our system. Without our body's miraculous processing systems for handling these dead cells, our life spans would be considerably shorter.

Colds, coughs, fevers and flus are healing processes

Although these conditions are usually referred to as "diseases," this is only because of the discomfort they cause as a result of wastes and toxins accumulating in the body and mildly poisoning it. For thousands of years it has been customary to refer to any abnormal feeling or state of the body as a disease. This custom considers only "what" and not "why" the body is experiencing this discomfort.

How can there be a cure for something that is not a disease? How can one cure something that is a normal body healing reaction? Why would one want to use any treatment, drug or antibiotic to stop the body from releasing the harmful effects of body pollutants?

From a simplistic perspective, colds, coughs, fevers and flus are "spring cleaning jobs." They are the body's emergency detoxifying processes for flushing out excesses of waste, pollutants, poisons and toxic residues that accumulate in the course of a year.

Just like any well-organized community, our bodies contain organs specially constructed to function as scavengers, waste disposals, conversion or recycling services, garbage dumps, garbage trucks, incinerators, and sewer pipes.

Forty percent of all waste management is handled by the liver. The intestines, kidneys, lungs, and skin flush out the remaining sixty percent. The thyroid is a thermostat that activates temperature increases to burn up (by fevers) body toxins. The thymus and lymph glands control the flow of poisons through lymphatic channels (sewer pipes). For any increase in retained toxins and body wastes to occur, one or more of these organs will not be functioning at their optimal efficiency.

People do not "catch" colds.

Infectious diseases are not evil witches

Colds, fevers and flus are NOT diseases. They are not causes of fever. Nor, as is commonly believed, are they caused by viruses and bacteria. Bacteria, viruses and fungi are not harmful agents flying randomly here and there, attacking unsuspecting victims, without reason or cause. Their primary purpose and role is always beneficial. They do not decide on their own to multiply into huge numbers, nor to mysteriously attack some innocent unsuspecting body, draining out energies and leaving the body almost helpless with aches, pains, lung spasms, and/or burning with fever.

Fevers, colds and flus are normal body functions

These conditions are defense mechanisms. They are emergency elimination and detoxification procedures which the body automatically brings into play whenever it experiences abnormal excesses and stagnating accumulations of body wastes, toxins, pollutants and poisons. They are the body's most effective means for protecting itself against potential harm that could be caused by retention of these toxins.

Normal body resistance and defenses

We are miraculously endowed with many organs and biochemicals which serve to protect us against excesses, wastes, infections and poisons. In a healthy body, miraculous, unerring processes immediately react to all pollutants and hazards. They trigger the body defenses to destroy, neutralize, oxidize, break down and eliminate everything that is not beneficial. This defense system successfully attacks every type of natural poison. It even struggles to protect us against man-created atrocities (pesticides, dioxides, PCBS, carcinogens, radiation, etc.).

Bacteria, fungi and viruses

All microbes are normal to the body. They are a natural part of the healthy body's defense team that performs regular detoxification processes. Microbes contain and secrete enzymes that digest, break down and destroy foreign abnormal molecular substances and detoxify them so they can then easily be eliminated.

All microbes are scavengers. Contrary to common belief, like bacteria they have an important beneficial function. Bacteria are irrepressible health protectors. They are not antagonistic, destructive, poisonous little beasties that must be annihilated by antibiotics at the first sign of their presence.

Bacteria, fungi and viruses can be compared to flies. One never finds millions of flies aggregating in one area unless there is a manure pile. Likewise, bacteria cannot grow unless they have rotting wastes to feed on. Infectious microbes only flourish when a body is already overloaded with toxins.

Microbes only grow when disease is already present. When they proliferate to excess, they begin to produce their own toxins and wastes. These are dumped into the body fluids and tissues and set off body reactions in the form of colds, fever and the flu. *They are not the primary cause of disease.*

As a part of the miraculous construction of our body and its built-in protective systems, our cells create their own bacteria, fungi and viruses. This process occurs when the cells die. The cell sacs or outer membranes collapse and the cell substance, or protoplasm, is dumped into the surrounding fluids. This leaves the membrane of the cell nucleus unprotected and exposed. Finally the nucleus also succumbs to destructive influences—toxins and waste.

At this point, the DNA and RNA of the chromosomes become vulnerable to the denaturing effects of the same toxins and poisons. These poisons either fracture the long chains of chromosome molecules or they combine with the chromosome fragments and trigger the formation and/or growth of long molecular chains. Based on the length/size of the chains or fragmented molecules created, they are called bacteria, viruses or fungi.

Illness is in the body long before a person experiences symptoms of disease and fever. All bacteria normally grow and feed on body wastes and poisons. Just as in nature, they act as scavengers that digest, break down and destroy body wastes, poisons, and foreign toxic elements in the body.

In a sense, bacteria and viruses can be compared to flies. When garbage builds up anywhere, inevitably it will attract millions of flies. Are flies the cause of garbage? Bacteria and viruses cannot grow in the body unless they also have a pile of rotting garbage and body wastes upon which to feed. **Accumulation of body wastes and toxins is always the cause of all fevers.** The body builds an internal bonfire (fever) to burn up the poisons.

Bacteria and viruses have a metabolism of their own and they function just like other living things. They feed on and digest excesses of their normal foods: the body toxins and accumulated wastes. This process of eating and processing toxins and waste is the reason for their existence in the body economy.

Like all living beings, they eliminate and excrete their own body wastes. Bacterial excretions are toxic. Whenever a fever-associated disease occurs there is always an excessive growth and build-up of microbes with their harmful excretions. It becomes important to prevent this microbial growth and secondary toxic build-up. One can accept that microbes of all kinds are causes of disease. However, **they are always only secondary causes.**

Most of us are unaware of the frauds perpetrated by the food industries that saturate and mummify foods with many poisons, preservatives, coloring agents, synthetic flavors, artificial sweeteners, emulsifiers, food stabilizers, softeners, thickeners and multiple other chemicals. Insecticides, hormones, antibiotics, chemical fertilizers and weed killer residues are present in most so-called healthy foods that are beautifully displayed on supermarket shelves.

Approximately two to three thousand chemicals are currently and commonly present in our daily diet. A great percentage of these are known as contributing causes of cancer. An even larger percentage has not yet been tested to determine the degree of hazard they present to the body. Unless we are highly selective about the foods we buy and eat, unconsciously we poison ourselves daily.

To these poisons add the stale, dead, devitalized and decaying overcooked, pressure or microwave "cooked"' and boiled or "fried to death" foods in our diet. Not only do we supersaturate our bodies by our intake of poison and junk; we also retain these foods and decaying remnants inside our intestines for unduly long periods of time. We are taught to naïvely believe that one bowel movement a day can be enough to eliminate amounts of daily ingested foods two and three times greater than stool bulk.

Since the average person in America has one bowel movement daily, both the medical profession and general lay public believe this is normal. This is adequate to keep the body cleaned out even from excessive food intake. It can keep the body free of toxic build-up from stagnating feces.

What goes into the body must come out. The amount coming out must obviously correspond to the amount that goes in.

Stresses, tensions, pressures, angers, resentments, hatreds, anxieties, fears and all other negative emotions and attitudes that constantly surround us and saturate our environments distort body chemistry and create toxins in the form of chemicals that are enormous threats to our health.

Our bodies are saturated by all these poisons, yet we naïvely believe there is no reason for illness, even if we live in a highly toxic environment. If illness "accidentally" occurs, a simple vitamin or mineral from a health store or a drug from a doctor will restore health.

Even a toxic body that is depleted and deficient still knows better. It will still protect itself against our abuse and ignorance. Our cells will create viruses, bacteria and fungi that have the ability to destroy our excesses and poisons.

Fevers are part of the body's defense process
Body wisdom creates fevers as part of its defense process. Whenever the garbage heap of body pollution piles up beyond a certain point, other body defenses take over to protect themselves. We bring on this defense system by excesses and indulgences coupled with failure to exercise enough—especially failing to perform the exercise of pushing ourselves away from heavily laden tables of food.

Colds are a similar body reaction
Colds are the result of a milder state of toxic accumulation. The body adequately rinses and flushes out these toxins by dissolving them in excess amounts of mucus secreted by the lungs, nose, sinuses and other tissues. The fluids ("catarrh") dissolve toxins and transport this waste from the body.

A special kind of cold is triggered by sitting in drafts or cold areas; we develop a "chill." Coldness stimulates over-activity of the thyroid gland. This gland produces an excessive amount of heat to compensate for increased body needs. In the process it also increases body metabolism. All body functions speed up with this increased heat production. Excess heat affects cells. The cells wear out and die much faster than normal. Cell breakdown releases excessive amounts of histamine and toxins into the tissues. These toxins and histamines create the symptoms known as flu or cold.

Antihistimines are the remedy of choice when getting a chill-type cold

If taken quickly, antihistimines can abort a cold in a very short period. It is advisable to use a non-drug form of antihistamine such as "Antronex" or "Antipyrexin" from Standard Process Laboratories of Milwaukee.

If taken early enough, one or two tablets are usually all that are required for relief. If taken after 24 hours from the time the cold symptoms appeared, antihistamines will have very little effect.

Flus are a method of body's defense against toxins

Flus occur from an unusual decrease or breakdown of one of the specific body resistance factors that allows or favors excess proliferation of viruses. The specific resistance factor is known as "phospholipids."

Phospholipids are normally found in soybeans and eggs. In its most concentrated form it occurs in lecithin.

Hangovers

A hangover is a period of reaction against alcohol, drugs, chemicals, and even body poisons. It is a "healing crisis" or "elimination crisis." There are no cures for hangovers. There is no cure for a cold.

Managing Colds, Flus and Toxins

Excess toxins and body wastes can build up in the body by excess intake from outside the body, or by breakdown of protective sacs that act as body storage areas. In either case, poisons flood the bloodstream and bring on the strong body reactions.

The healing processes and improved state of health that result from following a good health restoration regime will cause the storage area walls to collapse. The body will flush out residues of disease, toxins and body wastes piled up over the years.

If we have a history of many years of abuses and excesses along with constipation and faulty elimination, we may develop colds, fevers and flus—even following a healthy pattern of living that includes wellness therapies.

Patients who work hard and carefully follow a regime corresponding to their body needs yet become aware of a cold, flu or fever developing, will wonder why this occurs. Actually they are to be congratulated that their body has reached a level of health capable of attacking diseases and toxic storage places it couldn't handle before. They can still benefit from the same prescriptions described below.

All help provided to the body must be directed toward causes of the cold, fever and flu symptoms. Those causes are accumulations of body toxins, wastes, and pollutants.

All therapy should assist and intensify body mechanisms of self-defense and resistance to the poisons as well as to the microbial growth. Germ destruction is a normal function of the body. It does not require antibiotics or any other assistance except when the normally powerful body defense mechanisms are broken down, or when the body is in an emergency state. Its own resistance and bacterial agents of destruction are more effective than antibiotics and are completely harmless, without the side effects of drugs.

Some of these defense mechanisms are:
- **White blood cells -** Their normal function is to digest and break down all foreign elements in the bloodstream, including microbes.

- **The liver -** The main laboratory in the body for breaking down chemicals, poisons, unused, undigested food surpluses, and body wastes. It handles about 40% of all body putrification and transports poisons from the body by means of its carrier agent, called bile. Bile passes through the gall ducts into the intestines.

- **The Intestines -** Bowel movements eliminate wastes and poisons. Proper elimination three times a day is important for managing detoxification needs.

- **The Kidneys -** Water soluble toxins and minerals are soluble in the urine. They are flushed out through the kidneys.

- **The Thymus Gland -** Builds resistance and immunity to infection and toxins and stimulates the production of white blood cells. The thymus controls and intensifies elimination through the lymphatic channels, which are the body's sewage system.

- **The Lymphatic System -** Provides drainage channels to every cell and other area of the body. When not overloaded or blocked, it drains off excesses of body wastes and poisons and keeps the body clean and healthy.

- **The Spleen** - A filter of blood poisons and a blood rebuilder.

- **The Thyroid** - Increases body temperature whenever a fever is required to burn up wastes/residue that the body is not successfully handling in other ways. This process is like burning up garbage by means of a large bonfire.

- **The Lungs** - Toxic gasses and end products of the body's breakdown of poisons are flushed out through the lungs. They manage about 10% of body elimination.

- **The Skin** - Perspiration carries off toxic minerals and water soluble toxins. This process accounts for 10% of body elimination.

- **Body Acids** - 90% of the bacteria that trigger fevers and infectious conditions of the body cannot live in an acidic environment. Viruses may grow more favorably in an alkaline environment and require acid antagonism. *See cold therapies below.*

- **Excess alkaline wastes** - Fatigue or alkaline poisons; create a favorable environment for microbial growth and fevers.

- **Stomach secretions of acids** - An intake of acid food (vinegar, grains, oils and proteins) creates a resistance to bacteria and microbial growth.

- **Vitamin C** - Its ascorbic acid components are powerful microbial inhibitors and control agents of fevers. They also aid the body's oxygen delivery to red blood cells as they pass through the alveolar capillaries.

- **Oxygen** - Breaks down many poisons and microbes by oxidizing them.

- **Calcium** - In foods or in food concentrates, stimulates and increases the formation of white blood cells in the bone marrow. These are then "poured" into the blood and act as blood scavengers during periods of toxicity, infection and fever.

Recommended therapies for colds, fevers and flus

Drugs and antibiotics are not "therapeutic." Rebuilding host resistance and body health by eliminating toxic excesses IS!

Here's how:

- **Fasting:** The quickest and most valuable way to eliminate toxins and restore health.

- **Exercise:** Valuable during colds (only) to increase blood and lymph circulation and skin elimination by perspiration. Avoid during fevers and the flu.

- **Rest:** Eliminates fatigues, tensions and toxins. Especially important during fevers and the flu. Intense activity and work during these times can pose a threat to health reserves, i.e., to the adrenal (stress) glands and to the spleen.

- **Vitamin C (only in a complete whole concentrate form):**

  In our polluted environment, it is almost impossible not to burn up more vitamin C than could be available in our daily food intake. In a complete form we receive the benefits of *all* the accompanying team members (enzymes, minerals, proteins, etc.) that work together with vitamin C, creating a powerful team. This is much more effective than many thousands of milligrams of ascorbic acid, the so-called "natural" vitamin C tablets.

With so many defense processes, it seems almost a wonder that one can even get a cold, cough, flu, or infection. The abundance of body defense mechanisms presented in this book is an answer to the generally accepted idea that "there is no cure for the common cold or flu." The reason is, of course, that colds and flus are not diseases but rather, demonstrations of the body's wisdom, i.e., its need to eliminate wastes and toxins in order to restore balance.

No disease requires a cure, but there may be plenty of lifestyle habits and approaches to one's self-care that may need a "cure."

Chapter 18

The Cholesterol Myth

T hroughout the ages nature has visited a variety of plagues on mankind. An ironic twist has occurred regarding today's scenario. For the first time, the pharmaceutical companies in league with conventional medicine have created a man-made epidemic.

Cholesterolphobia (fear of cholesterol)

"Cholesterolphobia" started when the drug companies discovered a drug which they claimed would lower cholesterol levels. Up until that time a cholesterol problem never existed. In order to sell this drug to the unsuspecting public, they fabricated stories and propaganda condemning cholesterol as an evil and a menace. It was a subtle enemy that was lurking to stab you in the back and undermine your health.

Shattering the myths

Fears have a far-reaching and often devastating impact on body wellness and function. Fears also impede the metabolism of cholesterol in the liver.

The only way to eliminate this insidious phobia is to dispense with the following 10 myths:

Myth No. 1: *Cholesterol is not needed by the body.*
This just isn't so. Cholesterol is a necessary part of every cell. It helps to produce sex hormones and digestive juices. It aids in the absorption of physiological oils. We could not survive without cholesterol.

Myth No. 2: *The only way the body obtains cholesterol is by consuming it.*
Not so. About 80 percent of cholesterol in the human body is produced by the liver. This explains why it is difficult to decrease blood cholesterol merely by following dietary measures. Altering our own genetically controlled internal metabolism is as difficult as trying to change the spots on a leopard.

Myth No. 3: *The more cholesterol we eat, the greater the amount in the blood.*
This is not totally true. Cholesterol metabolism is somewhat like the thermostat that

controls the room temperature of our home. Studies show that the more cholesterol consumed, the less the liver produces. The absorption of cholesterol decreases and the excretion of cholesterol increases. If the diet is low in cholesterol, the liver gets the message to produce increased amounts.

Myth No. 4: *A single blood test is an accurate way to determine the level of blood cholesterol.* It is a fallacy to place so much faith in laboratory results. Studies show that laboratories have reported results that are either too high or too low by as much as 15 percent. Erroneous results can cause either needless worry or a false sense of security. Several tests are normally required to obtain a reliable figure.

Myth No. 5: *Precise blood test results can predict potential occurrence of a coronary attack.* Not so. A coronary attack is brought on much more by stress, tension, lifestyle excesses and blood circulation problems than by cholesterol. Abnormal cholesterols and abnormal cholesterol levels only add to predispositions for a heart attack that already exist.

Myth No. 6: *Dietary cholesterol is the primary risk factor for coronary disease.*
Life isn't that simple. It's unrealistic to believe that only one factor is responsible for heart troubles (or for any disease).

Genetics, diabetes, hypertension, smoking, lack of exercise, inadequate fiber intake, high fat diet, obesity and advancing age are important risk factors.

Myth No. 7: *A low level of blood cholesterol precludes atherosclerosis (hardening of the arteries).* Not so. Dr. Michael DeBakey, the famous Texas heart surgeon, reports that 30% of patients that have a coronary by-pass have normal blood cholesterol levels.

Myth No. 8: *Similar blood cholesterol levels trigger a similar number of heart attacks.*
Not so. The cholesterol levels of some males living in Edinburgh and Stockholm are identical. However, the number of coronary deaths for the Scottish is three times higher than that of the Swedish.

Myth No. 9: *Eggs should be avoided, as they increase blood cholesterol and trigger atherosclerosis.* Nonsense. Healthy eggs are a good source of protein, iron, phosphorus and vitamin A, and are low in saturated fats. It's prudent to have a varied diet. Blaming hens and cows for coronary disease is like accusing the iceberg of sinking the Titanic. A foolish captain sank this ship, just as surely as a heart attack results from a faulty and foolish lifestyle.

Myth No. 10: *Multinational chemical and drug companies have your well-being at heart.* You are being naïve and live in a "Never, Never Land" if you believe this one. Corporations deceive consumers in many ways. Some companies advertise their products as "cholesterol free" when, in fact, at no time did they ever contain any.

They load their products with sugar and salt, additives and preservatives. (Many foods that don't contain cholesterol create biochemical conditions in the body, causing cholesterol levels to increase.)

Research on cholesterol shows that:

- There is no relationship between the amounts of cholesterol and saturated fats you eat and incidence of heart disease. (Eskimos eat huge amounts of fats.)

- 80% of heart patients have normal cholesterol levels.[10]

- There is no scientific proof that lowering blood (normal) cholesterol levels prevents heart disease.

- There is no relationship between blood cholesterol levels and the degree of hardening of the arteries.

- Homocystene, not cholesterol, is the major cause of hardening of the arteries. Homocysteine is a toxic substance regularly produced from methionine. It remains toxic if not converted to cystethionine by the action of vitamin B-6. Vitamin B-6 is plentiful in fruits and vegetables; it is low in meats and dairy products.[11]

- High blood cholesterol levels are not acceptable or reliable predictors of heart or other disease risk. Blood cholesterol levels vary greatly, even throughout the day. Simply varying the positions of the body when blood is taken can alter test findings.[12]

  At best, blood cholesterol levels are only a crude indicator of many different diseases.

- Complications of high blood cholesterol are related only slightly to the amount of high quality food intake. Increasing food intake does little to increase blood cholesterol levels.

- Cholesterol is one of the essential building blocks of blood.

Misinformation about cholesterol

In order to convince the public that there is a cholesterol problem—one that can be serious that will probably require drugs for controlling it—food cartels and drug companies mislead us to believe that cholesterol and oils are harmful substances. This creates fear in the minds of an unsuspecting public that doesn't understand health and body physiology. Food and drug industries condition people to avoid the foods they need.

---

10 Framingham report, 1970 ... Drs. W. Kannel and T. Gordon.
11 Dr. K. Mccully, Howard Medical School.
12 Report from *The American Family Physician*, Sept. 1986.

Their advertising influence people to substitute cheap, counterfeit synthetic, instant, refined, attractively packaged, artificially or sweet flavored, phony "foodless" foods without cholesterol, for nourishing *whole foods* that contain quality oils. (They are performing one service in discouraging the purchase and use of the hydrogenated and rancid oils.) These commercial, refined and processed "non-cholesterol" foods are far more harmful than quality cholesterol foods. They upset and block the body's abilities to effectively utilize cholesterol.

Multiple warnings by the drug company-supported media against the ingestion of dairy products, eggs and butter deserve attention when they dissuade people from eating poor quality, unhealthy oil and fat foods.

It is misleading to consider all dairy products unhealthy or related to cholesterol issues.

It is perfectly fine to include dairy products in your diet if:
- They come from healthy animals and are used while still fresh.

- The animals have been fed with only quality foods, or chose their own foods in the fields, according to their needs. The feed given to these animals have not been contaminated with chemicals, drugs, or pollutants.

- The fields from which the animals choose their feed have not been contaminated by pesticides and chemical fertilizers.

- The animals have had no drugs, antibiotics, or hormones.

- The dairy products consumed are healthy and untouched by commercial and chemical processes—including pasteurization.

Most quality foods that are naturally rich in cholesterol also contain high levels of all the enzymes and chemical agents the body normally uses in order to metabolize and burn up excess cholesterol.

People are not informed that excesses of normal cholesterol are readily carried by the bile from the normally functioning liver to the intestines, which then automatically excretes them.

There is no real (high) cholesterol problem!
On the contrary, there can be problems of low blood cholesterol.

Low blood cholesterol health problems
Excess cholesterol is less of a problem than a deficiency. **Without cholesterol, the body could not live 30 seconds.** That's how important it is to our health and well-being. The quantity of cholesterol required by the body is second only to proteins and calcium.

Low blood cholesterol levels increase incidences of cancer, gall bladder problems, aggressive and violent behavior, homicide, suicide, personality disturbances, irresponsibility and poor self-control. They also accelerate body aging.

Stirring up our awareness of cholesterol may be a good thing, for it has alerted us to some far more serious and insidious problems regarding toxic fats, toxic oils and abnormal toxic cholesterol.

In chemistry books, oils are often referred to as "unsaturated fatty acids," causing confusion between oils and fats. "Unsaturated fatty acids" is a chemical term only. Oils are not fats and are as different as wood from steel.

Problems associated with faulty utilization/metabolism of cholesterol

A problem with cholesterol is comparable to a fire in which the wood doesn't burn properly, or to a car engine in which the gas does not completely ignite. In fireplaces and cars, the complications are carbonization; in people, it is hardening of arteries.

Main factors that hinder cholesterol metabolism and utilization are:

- Deficiency of vitamins and minerals (markedly affects and blocks cholesterol metabolism). These include: magnesium, potassium, manganese, vanadium, chromium, zinc, selenium, vitamins C, E, B-3, B-6 and Folic Acid.

- Deficiency and low intake of quality oils. Oils are tools needed by the cholesterol processing organs in order to metabolize the cholesterol. These oils—essential to good nutrition and necessary for the organs that metabolize cholesterol—are unavailable in a healthy form in grocery stores.

- Pre-packaging oil rich foods for quick use. Such foods, like roasted nuts, crushed cereal grains, and seeds, deteriorate quickly. Their oils are rancid before we buy them.

- An absence of enzymes required to properly and completely utilize (metabolize) oils and cholesterol. Pancreatic enzymes are the most important of these, since their role is to complete the digestion of oils in rich foods and make the oils available for absorption and use by the body.

With a pancreas problem, one can use Gamma-linolenic Acid (GLA for short). This oil does not need pancreatic enzymes to complete the body's digestive process. It is found mainly in borage seed, black currant and primrose.

Factors that play a major role in hindering the body's ability to utilize and burn up cholesterol and fats:

- Stress, tensions.

- Exhaustion, fatigue, burn-out.

- High sweets and sugar sources in the diet.

- All carbonated and alcoholic beverages.

- Tea, coffee, chocolate beverages.

- Cigarette smoking.

- Inadequate, incomplete digestion of fats/oils; insufficient pancreatic enzymes.

- Inadequate exercise (exercise releases tension).

- Faulty or inadequate functioning of body organs, eg., the liver and endocrine system.

Chapter 19

Denaturing of Oils and Fats

Oils become toxic in only one of two ways:
1. By natural processes
2. By commercial chemical processes

Denaturing nature

Seeds, cereal grains and nuts must be crushed or pressed in order to make oils readily available and create market appeal for cereals, nuts and nut butter. These oil rich foods have a hard outer coating. Nuts have hard shells. It takes a lot of pressure to break the outer coatings or shells and crush the kernels inside. Pressure creates heat. As the outer shell or coating of the oil containing food is broken, both the high temperatures of the press and exposure of the crushed material to the air allow the oxygen in the air to make contact and react with the oils. This causes the extracted oils in those foods to turn rancid. Rancidity can be identified by its foul taste and odor.

All oils go rancid. When they become stale, they turn rancid. Some oils, for example, wheat germ and flax seed oils, become rancid within days.

Toxic effects of rancidity:

- Rancid oils prevent the normal utilization and metabolism of cholesterol.

- Rancid oils are the most toxic of all foods. Even body wastes and excesses that get stored in fats are not nearly as toxic as rancid oils. The only substances more toxic and harmful are chemicals and drugs. Fats, chemically processed fats, lard, Crisco and shortenings, are also classified under the same rancid/toxic category.

- Stale rancid oils, like fats, interfere with and block the promotion of health and health-protecting functions of normal oils. They use up the place of normal oils in the body.

- Rancid oils block normal body oils from becoming transformed into hormones. When rancid, oils are no longer absorbed into the substances of the cell membranes. Cells lose their protective coating against environmental chemical hazards. The rancid oils then harm and poison cells.

- Rancid oils block the function and healing powers of our oil soluble vitamins.

A Commercial Answer to Rancidity

The food industry developed a process called "hydrogenation," which substitutes hydrogen for oxygen in order to avoid the foul taste and odor of oxygenated oils. Hydrogen combines with oils in the same way as oxygen. Hydrogenation is used for creating margarine, creamy peanut butters and various dressings and spreads.

Hydrogenation is artificial "rancidity." The hydrogen-processed oils have no foul rancid odor or foul taste. This fools the public into believing the oils they are buying and using are still fresh and of good quality. *The fact is, hydrogenated oils are just as toxic as oxygenated oils.* It makes no difference whether the oils are denatured by hydrogen or oxygen. Both denatured products create body toxicity.

Hydrogenated oils and fats are rich in abnormal, denatured cholesterol. They intensify the cholesterol problem, hinder the production of normal hormones and deprive the cells of their protective coatings.

Chemical Denaturing

Some chemicals react in ways similar to oxygen. Preservatives, foods additives, pollutants and drugs act on and denature oils in ways equal to or worse than those of oxygen rancidity or hydrogenation.

The worst enemy of oils is chlorine and members of the chlorine family. Chlorine bleaching is chemical oxidation.

Chlorine bleach destroys the foods or substances that cause stains; it attacks foods, oils and cholesterol. The amounts of chlorine in our drinking water are sufficient in concentration to do this.

Fortunately chlorine evaporates. When chlorinated water is allowed to stand in a jug on a counter, within 24 hours the chlorine has gone.

In our commercial foods, currently one can find up to 3,000 chemicals, additives and preservatives. Preservatives are food embalming substances. One can find many more in our polluted air and waters.

Even science doesn't completely know all of the chemical reactions that take place in our bodies, i.e., which foreign substances or pollutants are reacting with our oils and cholesterol. However, many scientists are surely aware that it is not possible for two incompatible chemicals to encounter each other without a reaction taking place. Any and all abnormal chemicals have an affinity for enzymes. When you destroy the enzymes that are part of the oil complexes, you destroy the ability of those oils as well as our cholesterol to function in their normal health giving ways.

Toxic oils excesses

It is almost impossible to find quality oils in ordinary grocery stores. Oils in the forms of standard salad oils and dressings, peanut and nut butters, sandwich spreads and similar foods are all chemically treated, hydrogenated, or rancid.

The following sources of fat toxicities are just as toxic, contribute just as much to our health problems, and thus are to be carefully avoided:

- **All commercially fried and deep fried foods** - French fries, corn and potato chips, fish-and-chips meals.

- **All pork products** - Ham, bacon, pork sausages, etc. Most pork foods can contain up to 50% fat (toxins).

- **Fats** - Are in the animal tissue cells that store body wastes, toxins and poisons. Unlike oils, they do not melt at body temperatures.

- **Fatty and greasy foods and fats of meats** - Duck and goose.

- **Margarines** - The harder the margarine, the more hydrogenated the oils; this includes soy margarines sold in health stores.

- **Coconut oils, and foods and candies made with coconut oil** - These foods are high in saturated oils. Oils that are available in grocery stores are usually rancid or chemically prepared.

- **Crisco, shortening, lards, and cooking fats.**

- **All oils that have been used for cooking** — These get heated at high temperatures. Never cook twice with the same oil.

- **Cotton Seed oils** - Are usually high in DDT.

- **Cream substitutes and artificial whipped creams; ice creams, sundaes, chocolate milks.**

- **Salted butter:** One never knows how long it has been stored; if stored too long it becomes rancid.

- **All processed, standard store-style sandwich spreads, margarines, and salad dressings.**

- **Oils packaged in clear transparent bottles -** Light rays can denature the oils as effectively as oxygen.

Defending oil against oxygen destruction

We breathe in up to fifteen hundred pounds of air daily. About 10% of this air (up to 150 pounds) is pure oxygen. It seems impossible to conceive that any substance in our blood or our bodies could escape from being oxygenated—especially our oils and oil soluble foods. The body has a protective barrier against the effects of oxygen. As anti-oxidants it uses alpha tocopherols, which are part of the vitamin E complex.

Toxic Fats

Fats are the body's storage tissues. They are deposit areas for wastes and excesses which the body cannot use, and for body poisons and toxins. This fat tissue is unhealthy and toxic. It is always a hazard to health.

In addition to serving as a good insulator against both hot and cold, fat tissue is a garbage pail for our normal body wastes. By storing these wastes, the fat keeps useless and hazardous substances from overloading the blood, creating congestion in organs, and interfering with normal healthy chemical reactions of body metabolism.

It is a serious mistake to confuse oils with fats. Fats contain little normal cholesterol, although they may store generous amounts of abnormal toxic cholesterols. Fats contribute more than any foods to high blood cholesterol levels.

Sources of toxic fats:

- **All prepared meats -** Salami, bologna, canned meats, hot dogs, sausages.
- **Red meats -** Even meats that appear lean have up to 18% fat. If eating meats, trim all visible fat before cooking.
- **Shellfish -** Clams, crab, lobster, oysters, scallops, shrimp. These are all high in cholesterol and lack the oils and enzymes for cholesterol metabolism.
- **Barbecued meats -** The overheated melted fat drippings are already rancid before they saturate the meats in the form of smoke, which is carcinogenic.
- **Canned tuna and salmon -** When these fish are fresh and have been prepared by broiling, their fats melt with the heat and can be poured off.
- **Sardines -** that are not packed in their own oil.
- **Gravies, sauces.**
  Commercial grocery store "assembly line" produced eggs - They are "sick" eggs. Sick eggs are sources of the greatest amounts of cholesterol. They lack normal lecithin and enzymes required by the body to use and

metabolize this cholesterol. Even a small number of sick eggs will add to blood cholesterol levels.

- **Butter rolls, commercial biscuits, donuts, sweet rolls, cheese breads, and commercial muffins.**

- **High fat cheeses, cream and processed cheeses.**

- **Milk and yogurt, and products made from these -** The fat content of skim milk may be tolerable, but the milk, especially if pasteurized, is not.

- **Cakes, pastries and other foods containing cooked commercial egg yolks.**

These factors foster cholesterol excesses in the blood and thus, are major health threats and causes of cholesterol related diseases.

Chapter 20

The Milk Myth

Do I really want to drink that milk??

From infancy we have been conditioned to believe that milk is a perfect food. We have been taught that it is wholesome and natural, that it's good for our health. Our mothers, our doctors and even our health departments have told us how wonderful it is.

Some people may hold these beliefs...others may not. Certainly researchers associated with medicine and the dairy industry who have thoroughly investigated every aspect of milk integrity have learned otherwise. Many medical research studies, enlightening reports from scientists in the milk industry itself and numerous studies from several countries by organizations similar to *Consumer Reports,* question the validity of our current beliefs about milk.

In this chapter we will discuss some of the findings that have been published in scientific journals. Our discussion will include data regarding side effects and commercial perversions of milk.

The fact is, milk is not as nutritious and beneficial as advertisements claim and want you to believe. Although the research findings presented here may seem comprehensive, actually they only touch the surface regarding information about milk.

Regardless of how convincing and impressive the advertising campaign and how convincing doctors, mothers and other authority figures have tried to be, it is our bodies—the benefits they receive or do not receive—that are the final judge.

A quality health-giving food must provide humans with all the nutrients essential to:
- Regenerate, repair and sustain body cells.
- Enable cells and organs, such as bones, nerves and teeth, to grow and mature normally.

- Sustain and balance body and mind functions.

- Resist diseases.

- Reproduce healthy and well-formed offspring.

- Provide energy, vitality, morale, and strength.

- Appreciate and enjoy the wonders of life and living.

Milk is or can be a good food only when it is:

- Whole—fresh from the cow.

- NOT pasteurized and NOT homogenized.

- From cows that are really healthy... which means they:
  - » Are not constantly immobilized in stalls.
  - » Are free to roam fields and maintain health and strength.
  - » Have been fed quality foods.
  - » Have never been treated with chemicals, antibiotics, drugs, hormones or Diethylstilbestrol.

- Ingested within hours after milking.

Hygienic care, quality diet and proper hormonal balance are as essential to the health of cows as for humans.

This presents three fundamental problems:

1. Cows used in large commercial dairy businesses are NOT healthy.
   A. Their diet and care do not and cannot sustain health.
   B. Only cows that have serious hormonal imbalances can produce large milk quantities and are used for milking.
   C. Inhuman care leaves the cows toxic and sick.

2. Even high quality milk directly after milking undergoes serious deterioration when subjected to all the commercial processes of handling.

3. Government and dairy industries have teamed up to make it illegal to obtain healthy and unpasteurized milk.

Mother's milk is the most perfect food for infants. There is simply *no* substitute that can provide so much high quality nutrition.

The charts below illustrate some of the main values of and differences between mothers' and cows' milk:

Composition of:	Cow's Milk	Mother's Milk
Acid/alkaline pH	Acid	Alkaline
Proteins	levels = 3 x higher than human needs. Difficult to digest	Quality and kinds needed are easier to digest by humans
Casein	80 – 90% of total	30 – 40% of total
Whey	18%	60%
Calcium	1250 mgms/100gms	118 – 340 mgms/100gms
Phosphorus	960 mgms/100gms	93 – 140 mgms/100gms
Milk Fats	3.7% = saturated Difficult to digest.	4.5% Fine emulsified Readily digestible
Galactose	High	High
Iron	Low	High 1mg/100gms
Zinc	Low	High
Pituitary (growth) hormones	Very high: enough to make a calf grow 600+ pounds in 1 year	Low: Proportioned to man's needs and bi-chemical balance. Approx 10 pounds child growth, 1st year

If you compare the mineral levels in human vs. cows' milk, you will discover significant differences between the two. In fact, the ratio of milk is different for every animal, suggesting the importance nature has placed on the different physiological needs of each animal on this planet.

Minerals in Human's and Cow's Milk (per 100 milliliters)

Element	Human Milk	Cow's Milk
Copper (mcg)	40.0	14.0
Iron (mcg)	100.0	70.0
Sulfur (mg)	14.0	30.0
Potassium (mg)	57.0	145.0
Chlorine (mg)	40.0	108.0
Magnesium (mg)	4.0	12.0
Calcium (mg)	35.0	130.0
Sodium (mg)	15.0	58.0
Phosphorous (mg)	15.0	120.0

Element	Concentration Range (milligrams/liters)
Zinc	0.4 – 8.0
Copper	0.15 – 1.34
Iron	0.20 – 1.45
Manganese	0.006 – 0.080
Chromium	0.00043 – 0.080
Selenium	0.007 – 0.06
Molybdenum	0 – 0.002
Cobalt	0 – 0.44
Nickel	0.01 – 0.15

The concentration differences viewed in these tables emphasize how necessary and important it is to recognize biochemical individuality.

All healthy unpasteurized milk contains and provides:

- **Galactose**
    - » Essential for the growth and integrity of the brain and nervous system. It is also a protective factor against multiple sclerosis.
    - » Provides protection against bacteria, tuberculosis, and leprosy.
    - » Antibody; provides immunity and antigen development for all body cells against viruses, flu's, AIDS, etc.

NOTE: *Galactose is destroyed by heat and fermentation of the milk; it requires lactase for its utilization.*

- **Antibiotics -** Protects the drinker from infections.
- **Calcium -** For bones, cartilages, ligaments, nerves, and teeth.
- **Phosphorus -** Indispensable for body utilization of calcium.
- **Ideal amounts of growth and healing hormones -** For those with inadequate production of pituitary hormones, an excellent medicine and supplement.
- **Valuable medicinal properties -** Increases and accelerates healing when the body's abilities are depleted.

Even with all these nutrients and properties, healthy unpasteurized milk presents significant problems:

- Biological and metabolic needs of humans and all animal species differ vastly. Nutrients for one species are never completely right for those of another, nor are they completely adaptable.
- It is not a question of whether milk is good for us; rather, it is a question of *whether the milk of an animal is good for a human.*
- No food has value to the body unless and until the cells completely utilize it.
- Milk can only be as healthy as the cows that create it. The body can only be as healthy as the food that goes into it. Putting diseased food into the body obviously causes diseases. It is important to drink and eat only healthy foods.

Many of the challenges of commercial milk are due to the following practices:

- **Cow Immobilization:** Commercial milking cows are imprisoned in their stalls and immobilized for days—weeks, by "neck bars." They experience restricted circulation and develop sicknesses that were formerly the plight only of humans.

- **Cow Feed:** Cows are what they eat. Profit motive restricts quality of cow feed to the cheapest, most inferior and least healthy. This feed filters through their body systems to their udders and into the milk, which then goes into, and affects our bodies. Much or most cow feed and consequently milk, contain varying amounts of the following:

  » **Cow Dung -** In many areas of the country cow dung is a normal, legally accepted portion of cow feed, used as a source of their protein intake.

  » **Pesticides and Chemicals -** Cow feed is commonly saturated with chemical fertilizers and pesticides from the grasses cows eat and that are used to treat most pasturelands. These readily saturate animal flesh and filter through and into the milk.

  » **Antibiotics and Drugs -** Poor feeding practices result in poor health and leave commercial milking cows so prone to infection, adding antibiotics to their feed becomes common and imperative.

  » **Hormones -** Excess secretion of pituitary hormones greatly increases milk production and money profits. DES, (Diethylstilbestrol) a synthetic pituitary-imitating-hormone increases milk production.

However, hormone imbalances whether from heredity or from any excess intake, can cause imbalances of all the other hormone glands. This means imbalance of hundreds of thousands of biochemicals that constitute body composition and function. Balance is the major factor in health. Biochemical imbalances are a major part of disease(s).

Pituitary hormones are growth hormones. Excess intake of DES predisposes and contributes to cancer.

- **Radioactivity**: Possibly a major number of milk producing cows feeds on alfalfa. Alfalfa is a plant that absorbs the largest amount of the chemical fertilizer potash.

  Potash is potassium that is mined. Potassium is a member of the radium-strontium family. It is about 50% as radioactive as radium. Radioactive cow feed turns into radioactive cow flesh and also radioactive milk.

- **Disinfectants:** Bacteria tend to multiply while milk is in storage.

- **Preservatives**: Chemicals are added to the milk to minimize bacterial growth.

NOTE: Freezing fresh milk would provide the same bacteria control and milk preservation. This costs more but would allow dairy farmers to by-pass the big dairy business. The dairy monopolies won't allow either.

- **Detergents:** Milking, cream and cooling equipment are washed with powerful detergents. No rinse is used after the detergent because water is supposedly a germ carrier. A high residue of detergent is left in the milk.

The health hazards just listed are made worse by transportation. In the trucks that deliver milk to the dairies, the healthy milk from healthy cows gets mixed together with: 1) milk from unhealthy cows, 2) milk contaminated from unclean udders, 3) barn dung, 3) pus and 4) other contaminants.

Milk destruction by pasteurization and homogenization

The purpose of milk pasteurization is to control and kill harmful bacteria by high heat. Pasteurization creates many side effects.

The high temperatures destroy valuable nutrients:

- **Proteins -** High heat denatures up to 90% of all proteins. Heated denatured proteins are useless as foods. Denatured proteins are like unnatural foreign substances in the body. They can be irritating, even hazardous, and worse still, a contributing factor to cancer.

- **Casein -** Cow's milk contains more than twice as much casein as human milk. This surplus is undesirable and difficult to digest, especially for babies. The heat of pasteurization transforms casein into percaseinae, a perverted substance that has a powerful chemical affinity for calcium. It combines with, binds, immobilizes and renders unusable all calcium molecules it contacts.

- **Lysine -** This protein is essential for:
  - » Growth and calcification of teeth and bones.
  - » Protection against cavities and arthritis.
  - » Assimilation of all other amino acids via the digestive tract.
  - » Stimulating secretion of gastric enzymes.
  - » Protecting the liver against cirrhosis; lysine is very susceptible to high heat and is destroyed and denatured by pasteurizing.
- **Mineral and Trace Minerals -** Minerals are the structural building and reinforcing elements of all body cells and organs. Trace minerals are the principle ingredients of all enzymes. They are indispensable catalysts for food utilization and body functions.

- **Calcium -** Cow's milk does not contain enough calcium to saturate the percaseinate thirst. The ingested percaseinate steals large amounts of calcium from the body.

  Only unpasteurized milk provides the body with the calcium needed for bones, nerves and teeth, etc.

  Pasteurized milk takes calcium out of the body.

- **Iron -** For both children and adults alike, iron is in readily assimilable form in the milk before it is pasteurized. After pasteurization it quickly precipitates into an unassimilable form. Demineralization that is hazardous to one's health can result.

- **Unsaturated Fatty Acids -** These raw materials are essential to the endocrine glands (ovaries, thyroid, sex glands, adrenals and liver) for manufacturing hormones that perform their normal functions. Up to 90% of these indispensable nutrients are destroyed and denatured by pasteurizing. The resulting denatured fats increase blood cholesterol.

- **Vitamins -** Anywhere from 10% up to 90% of all vitamins are destroyed by the high heat of pasteurizing. This adds to serious deficiencies. Vitamin destruction is increased by the action and effects of sunlight, oxidation and storage time.

- **Enzymes -** The body requires hundreds of thousands of enzymes to function or live. Enzymes work as teams in conjunction with vitamins. No health or body balance is possible unless all the enzymes are available and functioning. They are the essential agents that make possible every physical, mental, emotional biochemical function of healing, feeling, living, thinking, cell restoration, health maintenance; and neutralization and elimination of all poisons and body wastes. Like vitamins, enzymes must be constantly replaced and replenished. Living foods are their only source.

  Enzymes are not contained in or provided by common vitamin-mineral tablets or health store supplements. Raw milk contains many enzymes. The denaturing and destruction of these enzymes is the result of pasteurization (high heat), sunlight and oxidation, or contact with air.

- **Lactic Acid -** Lactic acid is destroyed by pasteurization. This important constituent of milk is an essential nutrient for normal bacteria of the intestines. The intestinal bacteria are responsible for breaking down fecal matter and maintaining bowel health. They also create the indispensable vitamin B complex.

- **Bacteria -** The primary purpose of pasteurization is to kill harmful bacteria in milk and make it safe and pure to drink. Although to a certain extent it achieves this temporarily, it also destroys the bacteria that manufacture lactic acid in the bowels. All milk, even fresh from udders, normally contains some bacteria. Milk itself fosters bacteria growth.

  » Healthy cows' milk has only as few as 50 bacteria per cubic centimeter—a negligible amount. This count can grow up to 50,000 bacteria per cubic centimeters in 24 hours, an amount acceptable by legal standards.

  » Bacteria levels of unhealthy cows' milk at the time of milking usually number up to 50,000 bacteria per cubic centimeters. Each day, bacterial growth can increase to levels of up to 500,000 live bacteria per cubic centimeters. It is illegal to sell all milk at these levels that is over 24 hours old.

» Pasteurizing reduces the 500,000 live, harmful coli bacteria contained in each cubic centimeter to 50,000 bacteria per cubic centimeter. This is barely within the legal limit of hygiene and safety.

» The 450,000 dead bacteria per cubic centimeter are not filtered out. This dead bacteria and their denatured proteins are still in the milk that is sold.

Milk pasteurization fosters the growth of bacteria

The pasteurizing heat destroys bacterial growth inhibitors (antibiotics) that are normally found in raw, unheated milk. The 50,000+ surviving, living bacteria feeding on denatured proteins and dead bacteria residues increase ten times in 24 hours. During this time the bacteria count is back up to 500,000 bacteria per cubic centimeters (500,000 live + 450,000 dead bacteria).

One million bacteria per cubic centimeters is much greater than the legally allowed health level. If one were to put a glass of 24-hour-old pasteurized milk through a filter, one-third of the amount in the glass would be solid bacteria. This is about the same number one would find in pus or excrement (*I apologize for the reference*).

With so many horrible side effects, why is pasteurization still legally imposed on all milk?

Originally pasteurization was a hygienic measure legislated to prevent tuberculosis and other bacterial plagues.

Why is pasteurization still required and in effect when according to government laws, we are assured that:

- All milking cows are constantly and thoroughly inspected for disease?

- The infectious diseases of the cows are thoroughly controlled by antibiotics and by many hygienic methods?

- All barns and environmental conditions in which the cows are kept are rigorously checked and controlled?

- All milking and storage conditions are hygienically inspected and controlled?

Homogenization

Like the word "pasteurized," "homogenized" suggests (falsely) that the milk has undergone yet another process for its improvement, i.e., for your benefit.

Homogenization mixes or combines the milk fat and milk. The fat droplets are pulverized and become extremely small. This makes it possible to create a stable suspension of fat in the milk. It becomes "homogenous."

Through this homogenizing process, the minute fat particles can now readily pass through the intestinal wall and into blood vessels. Via the blood they enter into the tiny network of capillaries that maintain a normal flow of blood and nourish the blood vessels.

Once inside the capillaries they form deposits of fat and cholesterol that clog the blood vessels' thread-like capillaries in various organs of the body, including the heart.

NOTE: Normal milk fat droplets are too large to do this.

These fat and cholesterol deposits can lead to hardening of the arteries and heart attack, mankind's most common killer.

Homogenization is also a process for treating stale, rotting milk. As bacterial growth becomes excessive, i.e., as the milk starts to turn sour (acid), the liquid separates from the rest of it, masquerading its staleness as freshness.

By adding a sodium or alkaline chemical, the souring of milk and bacterial growth are blocked. The acid is neutralized and normal milk flavor is restored. The milk is again drinkable and saleable. But is it healthy? Hardly.

The third purpose of homogenization is obviously to prevent milk losses and make money by deception.

POWDERED OR DRIED MILK
Two processes are used for preparing milk powder:
1. Spray drying - This process produces very little change in the milk's quality.
2. Superheating on metal surfaces - Superheating destroys and denatures many more proteins than the process of pasteurization. Much more lysine is destroyed (see previous comments about lysine). These hazards are intensified if and when the powder is stored for a long time.

   Most powdered milk is dried by superheating. Considerable amounts of milk are sold in what appears to be its original state. Appearances are deceive. It is reconstituted powdered milk.

Boiling Milk
Effects are similar to the superheating process but considerably more devastating than the effects of pasteurization. ***Never boil milk!***

With so many changes and so much denaturing taking place in milk, obviously milk drinking presents many hazards.

To preserve one's health it is most important to be aware of what denatured milk can do to the body's bones, teeth and nerves. It is also important to consider side effects of the chemicals, pesticides, fertilizers, radioactivity, animal diseases, bacteria, etc., found in milk that goes through normal processing before it reaches the grocery store.

Pasteurized cheeses and yogurt have similar side effects. Most cheeses, unless specially marketed in health stores or unless they are strong and aged over 90 days are pasteurized. Processed creamy cheeses are much more denatured and toxic than anything mentioned above. They can contribute to loss of immunity and predispose to cancer.

Following is a list of conditions caused by milk drinking and ingestion of milk products, or to which milk and milk products can be and often are an important contributing factor:

- **Lowering of body immunity:** Healthy milk normally contains and provides factors that protect against some diseases. These are destroyed by pasteurizing.

- **General body toxicity:** Overheated proteins are denatured and toxic. All of the antibiotics, pesticides, drugs, chemicals, chemical fertilizers and milk components destroyed by radiation, toxins of the cow's disease(s) that filter into the milk, and rotting bacteria, are toxic and add to the drinker's toxicity.

- **Eczema:** Skin breaks down under the influence of excess body poisons and wastes that exit through the pores. Usually a lack of skin oils, vitamin complexes and calcium render the skin more sensitive and prone to being damaged by the listed toxins and poisons.

- **Weakness, Fatigue:** Toxicity drains the energy from our bodies and leads to exhaustion. It is more taxing on the body systems than fatigue. One has only to have experienced food poisoning to be aware of this.

- **Mucus, Ear Aches, Colds & Flu's -** Denatured and toxic milk and milk products bring about the production of mucus by the mucus secreting linings of deferent organs, including the nose, lungs, sinuses, stomach and intestines, prostate gland and kidneys.

- **Sinusitis & prostate congestion -** These conditions are brought about by an overloading of catarrh[13] and body toxins. (See "Mucous" above)

- **Lung Congestion, Bronchitis & Colitis -** Mucus is a fluid secreted by surfaces cells of organs to protect themselves from toxins, irritants,

---

13 A disorder of inflammation of the mucous membranes in one of the airways or cavities of the body

denatured proteins, chemicals, drugs, etc. Mucus dilutes the poisons, serving as a flushing agent. It carries them out of the body.

- **Tonsillitis -** Tonsils are large lymph glands. They are the immune system's first line of defense against ingested or inhaled foreign pathogens. When they become clogged with toxins they aid in the process of disease.

- **Swollen Glands -** Mucous produced by milk thickens the fluids in the lymph ducts, whose role is to carry away the constant outpouring of cell wastes and toxins from tissues. Mucous from milk hampers lymphatic drainage, clogs glands, and retains poisons.

- **Allergies -** About 25 to 35% of infants are allergic to milk. Allergies are a condition resulting from the body's loss of ability to detoxify and eliminate irritants, toxins, poisons, etc.

The essential role of enzymes is to digest, absorb, use and eliminate nutrients and denatured substances in all foods, including milk. Anything entering the body that is not properly handled by the body's enzymes becomes a foreign substance and an allergen.

Pasteurizing milk causes enzyme destruction, one of many deleterious consequences.

Cows' milk allergy may seem to disappear as one gets older. This is a misconception. Although tolerance may develop over years, at a certain point the allergy will reappear.

> *"The main organs affected by allergies are the joints,*
> *the intestines, the blood vessels, circulation personality and behavior."*
> *—Dr. Stevan Cordas, D.O.*

Allergies often manifest in the following ways:

- **Lactose intolerance:** Lactose is a sugar that cannot be properly digested or utilized after the age of three. The enzymes for processing lactose are often depleted by that age. Every 8-ounce glass of milk contains about one ounce of lactose.

- **Asthma:** To a considerable degree, these are also allergy types of hay fever reactions.

- **Bloating**
  - » Indigestible lactose ferments in the intestines.
  - » Undigested, denatured proteins putrefy (rot) in the intestines.
  - » Both processes produce intestinal gas with bloating and swelling of the stomach.

- **Diarrhea:** Excess contracting of the intestines can occur when irritating, harmful, putrefying, undigested substances in food or milk are dumped into the intestines. Flushing or forcing these out of the body (diarrhea) is a normal protective reaction, therefore not to be considered distressful or treated and blocked by drugs.

- **Colitis Enteritis:** This condition results from constant irritation of the colon intestine by infiltrated milk substances: lactose, denatured proteins, pollutants, or added chemicals.

- **Constipation:** Many "old wives" over the centuries knew that giving boiled milk to infants stops diarrhea. Pasteurized milk can likewise hamper normal bowel elimination and cause constipation. It would therefore seem prudent to suggest that anyone who suffers from inadequate elimination should definitely stay away from commercial (pasteurized) milk.

- **Infant colic cramps:** Pasteurized milk is particularly harmful to babies as it tends to irritate the intestinal walls. Frequently it causes colic (intestinal cramps) and can cause pinpoint hemorrhages in the intestinal wall with slow oozing and loss of blood.

- **Calcium deficiency diseases:** The "percaseinate-bound" calcium can affect nerves, bones, ligaments and teeth. Lack of calcium decreases white blood cell production by the bone marrow. Evidence indicates that calcium problems contribute to and/or help to accelerate the following calcium related conditions:

  » Faulty growth of bones, nerves, and teeth in infants.
  » Nerve diseases: irritability, restlessness, nightmares, convulsions, epilepsy, nervous conditions, personality problems, lassitude, decreased ability to concentrate, multiple sclerosis, and nerve degenerative diseases.
  » Bones - Osteoporosis, Arthritis.
  » Teeth - Cavities, Jaw bone erosion, Pyorrhea.
  » Infections - Resistance to blood toxins and infections is an important part of calcium induced, increased production of white blood cells.
  » Arthritis - Streptococcus B is a bacteria sometimes found in milk and cheese that may cause rheumatoid arthritis. This bacterium is resistant to the heat of pasteurization.

- **Cancer:** Certain dairy products, such as cheese and especially cottage cheese, can be a precursor to breast cancer, benign breast lumps and chronic cysts. Cheese contains estradiol, a form of female hormone. Estradiol concentrates in excess can cause breast diseases.

- **Heart Attacks:** Milk fat contains Xanthine Oxidase, an enzyme that helps metabolize cholesterol and prevents its excess. This enzyme is destroyed by homogenization. Because of the calcium deficiency brought on as a result of percaseinate thirst (mentioned earlier), the vagus nerves can overactivate the heart muscles. This can cause heart muscle cramping with irregular and fast heart beats. Pressure from heart muscle cramps causes constriction and closure of the heart's blood vessels.

- **Stomach Ulcers:** Milk has been a standard medical treatment for ulcers, since it has the ability to neutralize stomach acid (hydrochloric acid). When the stomach is empty of food, hydrochloric acid erodes its inner skin and creates ulcers. Neutralizing this acid protects stomach acid from erosion.

  Drinking heated milk triggers the production of mucus and coats the stomach lining. The ulcers may not be healed but are simply protected and coated by mucus. Along with this relief comes a price: frequent intake of pasteurized milk fills the stomach with denatured and hard to digest protein molecules, indigestible lactose, chemicals, pesticides, rotting bacteria, etc. These pollutants irritate the stomach wall and trigger an increase in secretions of hydrochloric acid. The ulcer process is also perpetuated by milk consumption.

- **Headaches:** Tyramine, a breakdown product of casein, is an amino acid found in milk and cheese. Amounts present in dairy foods are both excessive and poorly tolerated by humans. It is a common cause of both migraines and high blood pressure.

- **Pregnancy problems:** The rate of unsuccessful pregnancies, still-births, premature births and miscarriages followed by complications greatly increases when expectant mothers consume large amounts of pasteurized milk.

- **Cheese problems:** Many of the above problems arise also from eating large amounts of cheese, which is merely fermented milk without its whey. Whey is high in casein and globulin.

When the milk industry, doctors and pseudo-nutritionists promote milk as the ideal food for health, we are led to believe that what is made available and sold to us as milk is *real milk*: natural milk that is health promoting, untouched, unhampered and undestroyed.

Big business promotes ways to create illusions that stale milk is still fresh and that pasteurized and homogenized milk still contain and provide health-creating nutrients. One cannot tell the difference by appearances and taste.

Once denatured by all the dairy industry processes and pasteurizing machines, milk undergoes biochemical changes and retains about as much of its nutritional identity and integrity as a brand new Cadillac after being hit by a bomb. The milk you buy today is about as natural as a soda drink or a synthetic food.

Since all of this information is well-known and has been validated by the milk industry and medical researchers, what reason could possibly exist for pasteurized, homogenized and stale milk to still be sold?

The answer to this question should be self-evident. The main purpose of the proponents of pasteurization and homogenization, and of those who make the laws for pasteurization is to promote long milk shelf life and sales… *profits*.

Their goal is not to produce healthy milk!

Changes resulting from pasteurizing and homogenizing:

- **Fat** - Changes in cream formation.
- **Lecithin** - Destroyed through splitting up of phosphoric acid.
- **Casein** - Heat changes casein into rennet and into an acid. Casein changes into percaseinate, which binds all milk calcium. This process makes it impossible for the body to use any calcium and even leaches it from the body.
- **Lactose** - This is milk sugar. It becomes caramelized.
- **Citric Acid** - Destroyed.
- **Soluble Calcium Salts** - Transformed into an insoluble, unutilizable form.
- **Carbonic Acid** - Destroyed.
- **Vitamins and Enzymes** - Practically all destroyed.
- **Antibiotic & Bacterial Properties** - Destroyed.
- **Vitamin C** - Destroyed.
- **Proteins** - Denatured, perverted. Up to 90% destroyed.

Anyone for a glass of milk?

Chapter 21

The Importance of Sleep

*At one time it was normal practice for the family physician
to prescribe bed rest for virtually any disease.*

Sleep is such a logical, natural and valuable healer, it makes one wonder why most doctors today usually ignore its benefits. Maybe because it's just too simple and easy to recommend, or maybe because it's just not scientific enough, i.e., chemically testable in a laboratory.

Could it be that sleep is such an effective remedy that it would eliminate or interfere with the need for many drugs—thus interfering with this powerful industry's bottom line profits?

Whatever the reason, sleep merits much more consideration and frequent use because **there is no health restoration without sleep!**

Sleep is:
- Slowing down of the body's activities, functions, metabolism and vibrations of living. Whenever a body wants or needs to heal, it switches itself to a state of rest and sleep or lowered vibrations. This is called the "alpha" state.

   It is as if the body does not have the power to be totally active and capable of repairing, regenerating and healing itself at the same time. It can do one or the other at any one time, but not both simultaneously.

- A chemical state. It is the role and function of alkaline minerals to slow down the body, help it to release tension, and relax. Sleep is a state of alkalinity for the entire body. Alkalinity is body sedation and preparation for sleep.

- The state of repairing all the wear, tear and used-up cells and materials from which they are constructed.

- The state of replenishing our cells' vital forces which have been burned up and depleted by all the activities of the previous day. Sleep restores energy reserves for the next day's activities.

- The condition our bodies use for healing. Health restoration and rebuilding take place only during periods of sleep and relaxation. Almost no healing occurs during daytime activity.

Sleepiness

When all the daily activities have used up your energy resources, your body tires out. You will feel tired and experience sleepiness; you will want to sleep.

Sleepiness is a great wellness detector that tells you to slow down, go back into low gear, relax, and sleep.

It is the body's way of telling the brain centers that control our living, that we need to replenish our energies and rebuild all the billions of cells that wore out, died, and now need to be replaced with new, vital, alert, vigorous ones. It is our time for health renewal. Sleep creates the conditions for healing and health.

The sleepiness you experience following normal days of activity may be more pronounced if you are following a health restoration or healing program. If you are attentive to your needs during any illness, your body will want to utilize everything you're doing in order to help it heal, and it will sink into a sleeping state. This sleep indicates that the regime you're following is good and is working for your benefit. Don't be concerned about being more tired than usual. You need the sleep. Live with it. Accept it and be content with it.

The Body's Healing Processes

Enzymes are in charge of all body healing and restorative processes. They are the keys to all healing. However, they act only when teamed with other biochemicals.

Their teammates are proteins, oils, minerals, trace minerals and vitamins. It is the team rather than the individual biochemical that is responsible for healing and other life functions.

Enzymes catalyze the joining or separating of special magnetic type bonds that "knot and tie together" the molecules.

During the daytime and periods of active living, these enzymes split the bonds and separate the bonding elements. Since all elements are held together by a great amount of energy, when the cells split, this energy is released—a process similar to atomic fission. The resulting energies are now available for organs, cells, and tissues.

Like motors using fuel, every part of our body uses this energy to perform its life functions.

During sleep, enzymes build new cells, tissues and body biochemicals. They perform this function by bonding all the necessary components, similar to cementing brick to brick.

This only happens when we sleep.

The state of our body's acidity or alkalinity signals to the enzymes whether they should bind molecules and rebuild the body, or split molecules and energize it. When the body is acid, the enzymes break bonds. When the body is alkaline the enzymes create bonds.

Insomniacs

Most people who believe they are insomniacs really are not. They may lie in bed for hours thinking they are constantly awake, and are not aware of the moments they sleep. Much of this "sleep" time may be dream-filled or gives one the impression of being awake.

The easiest mistake you can make during periods of wakefulness is to worry about not being asleep. Your eyes may be open, or you think they are. As you rest, the majority of your body and its faculties may be in a soporific state. This is adequate to regenerate and restore body and cell integrity.

Sleeping "like a log" is not normal, nor is it possible without the abnormally sedating action of drugs. Numerous times during the night while asleep, the body normally changes position. This is essential in order to prevent circulation stoppages by compression of the body parts that receive our weight when we lie on them. During changes of position one may momentarily sense awakening.

Sleep Deficiency

During difficult and tense periods of living—and even more so during periods of health restoration and healing—people need much more sleep.

Frequently repeated nights of insufficient sleep can accumulate like overdrafts in a bank account. They can bankrupt your health, your immunity and your body's ability to stave off disease, exhaustion and/or breakdowns.

Insomnia is a major contributor to aging. Normally with age comes a decrease in the pace of life. Mind-body activities decrease and we tend to make fewer demands on the nerves. We also experience less wear, tear, and acidity. The number of hours of sleep required to regenerate body and mind integrity normally should also decrease.

When unable to sleep:

- **DON'T** allow long hours of inability to sleep get you up-tight, concerned or upset. Developing a dread of sleeplessness interferes with your ability to sleep.

- **DON'T** be anxious if sleep doesn't come to you as you would like. This is counter- productive. One night without sleep depletes very little of your energy and life resources.

- **DON'T** fear being exhausted the next day. Your energies can be replenished. You can miss a whole night's sleep and experience as much well-being and energy as if you had experienced those hours of sleep, by taking special whole food concentrates that provide the total life force of the foods from which they are extracted.

- **DON'T** toss and turn restlessly. Let your body just be. Close your eyes. Breathe deeply and slowly. Let go. Relax.

- **DON'T** use sleeping pills, except as a last resort. Sleeping pills are for extremes of insomnia—the type that is brought on by severe trauma, shocks, losses and grief. These stresses impose an abnormal impact on the body and nervous system.

- **AVOID**
  - » Coffee, caffeine, and tea
  - » Chocolate, candies, bars and sweets
  - » Pep pills, diet pills
  - » High acid foods
  - » Soft drinks, diet drinks

Chapter 22

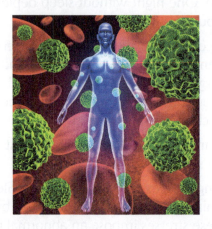

Cancer

Curing is not finding a doctor who will cure us,
but rather finding the "self" we have lost.

Dealing with cancer

If you have recently been diagnosed with cancer, you may be experiencing a wide variety of emotions: fear, anger, sadness, guilt, helplessness and anxiety. More often than not, you are faced with the hopelessness of what has long been believed and taught about cancer.

The experiences of millions of cancer victims and helplessness of their doctors is like a contagious disease that seeps into your thinking, feeling and morale. You've already learned about the tortures and pain that cancer patients can endure before passing away.

Under the circumstances, how can you approach your own condition except with the same discouragement of those who have died before you? How do you escape the panic and fear that doctors leave you with?

You are now faced with "what do I do"?
How do you change your life from disease to wellness? How do you get rid of all the causes and counteract their impact as they threaten to destroy your body and

your life? How do you rejuvenate and rebuild your body and life so you may "really" regain your vigor and hope for many future years of enjoyment free from disease and the horrors that disease can produce?

How can you be free from fear?

For centuries we have been conditioned to believe that nothing can be done for cancer except kill the cancer cells and tumors. We have been taught to see cancer as a formidable, mysterious, insidious disease and to accept it as a diabolical mysterious force that has no manifestation other than a tumor. We are told that our bodies are ignorant and helpless and there is nothing we as a patient can do—that our bodies have no wisdom of their own that would guide us back to health.

We have been given a message: "Don't think for yourself. Be a gentle and compliant soul. Whatever can be done must be done for you by doctors and hospitals. Go along with every treatment your sincere, good-hearted family physician, aided by the brilliant oncologist, has offered, even if it kills you (and it probably will)."

Conventional medicine has maintained that cancer is an invasion of the body from inside, by cells that have gone wild. It tells us that cancer cells are formed throughout life, but are normally detected and routinely destroyed by the body's immune system. Cancer develops when this system fails. Treatment consists of efforts to remove or destroy these malignant cells by surgery, radiation or drugs.

Where do such ideas you are expected to believe come from? Not from medical science or knowledge, but from the ignorance of many centuries.

To climb back up from the depths of your distress and reach the pinnacle of your human potential is a long and arduous path. If you want to reach the heights of health you will need clear vision of the road ahead. You will need to make changes in your thinking and learn to believe again in positive possibilities instead of negative dead end despair. You must fight the deceit and cunning of disease with positive awareness and strength of will. You are going to need encouragement as a healing weapon.

You must set aside the mindsets of helplessness or inadequacies the medical profession follows and offers to all of its cancer patients. In the following pages we will share answers that can relieve at least some of your anxieties. First and foremost, merely understanding the nature of cancer and why and how you got it can be a big help.

What is cancer?

Cancer is generally the result of a multitude of causes which over time have systematically broken down the body's immune system, compromised its resistance to disease and eventually built up an alternate defense system in the form of a tumor.

Cancer is like a number of diseases all attacking the body at the same time.

Tumors are not the cancer! They are only a part of the body's system of resistance to the many causes that threaten to perpetrate murder, with you as their victim.

The real disease is the sum total of all the body wastes and poisons, the highly toxic carcinogens and chemicals, severe deficiencies and forces that have accumulated over a period of many years. At a certain point they start to damage cells and their chromosomes, perverting and transforming them into rapidly growing abnormal ones and insidiously destroying our body's ability to detoxify, eliminate and defend itself against them.

When cancer causing toxic substances reach levels that are destructive to the cells, the body transforms damaged cells into millions of microscopic mini-sacs. It dumps as many of these virulent poisons as possible into the cell sac. The cells become storehouses for the cancer causing poisons. These storehouses are called "tumors."

When all other defenses fail, the best system the body can develop for protecting itself against chemical threats is to create a garbage disposal (tumor). Our body's higher wisdom takes over as it struggles constantly to protect every gland, organ and function from disease.

Removal of these poisons from the body's circulation is an ingenious life protecting strategy, for if these toxic wastes were to continue to circulate in the blood as it travels throughout the body, they would eventually destroy it.

Viewed in this light, tumors are important warriors in the body's defense system. They are red flags warning us that excesses of poisons are menacing our life. The real evil is the sum total of all of its causes: the cell destroying poisons, forces and abnormalities.

SIX POSITIVE PRINCIPLES FORM A BASIC STARTING POINT:

Read them carefully and think about them. Digest them with your mind. Learn to appreciate them and keep them foremost in your beliefs. Then use them. They are powerful weapons of healing.

1. **Realize and try to accept that having cancer does not mean you have to die**. It means you have to relearn how to live. In order for you to live your full, completely true nature, you have to take your life in your own hands and care for it. *Really care for yourself.*

2. **It is not possible for disease and health to coexist in a body at the same time.** Both states existing at the same time is a contradiction of

terms. If your total health could be completely restored, your disease must disappear.

3. **Your body knows infinitely more about healing itself than any scientist, doctor or healing professional.** Only your body knows what it needs in order to heal; it has the secret remedy. Therefore, seek your own body wisdom and not the ignorance of the past… not the books, someone else's body, or remedies that were beneficial to and effective for others. Do not seek treatment systems that destroy only tumors but do nothing to get rid of causes and nothing to rebuild resistance, healing and health.

Look into the world of your cells. Look into your mind, your emotions, your life, your values and your attitudes. Evaluate all deviations from normal. Check out and change everything that is not YOU, not supportive of you—contrary to and against your nature and your life purpose.

4. **Only your body has the ability to heal. Only bodies heal. Doctors cannot do this for the body.** Find out which of your healing abilities have been depleted. What nutrients, enzymes, proteins, minerals, vitamins, oils, life forces are missing? Provide your body with everything it needs.

   Also, it is essential to break down and eliminate any hindrances and barriers to healing. What are all the abnormalities in your life that are blocking your body from living in an optimal state of well-being?

   Believe that you cannot stop your body from replacing sick and dying cells with perfectly normal body cells. This is healing.

5. **It is not true that there is very little anyone can do for cancer other than kill tumors.** In fact, so much can be done, the real problem is figuring out which of many things can and should be employed, based on the patient's body and condition. It would take a small book to discuss all the possibilities of helping cancer patients. This is summarized later.

6. **You can't and won't die until you allow yourself to die—until you give up and want to die.** One aspect of our nature that stands above all others is our **free will**. Even the God who created us will not interfere or override this prerogative. If we refuse to give our lives back to Him, He does not argue or resist.

   Of course when whatever is required for our health and joy of living is depleted, destroyed or blocked from being a part of our nature and function, we lose our desire and readily beg for deliverance.

You are being asked to believe in your body, to believe there is innate body wisdom that is greater than science and medical technology. You are expected to believe that your body does not make mistakes. If it isn't making a mistake, you need to understand the reason for the body's manifestation of tumors, pain and disease.

Your perspective, how you view cancer and how all the causes relate to you—how you have contributed to bringing it to yourself—plays a major role in determining how you are going to embark on the pathway to restoring your health.

Believing in your nature, in your body's wisdom and healing abilities and in your role as healer, requires faith.

Your faith can make you whole. To restore health without faith is an impossible task. With faith, it is amazing what our bodies and minds can do. You need every ounce of these healing powers. If you cannot accept the common sense concepts we present here, you will have lost the support of powerful forces. Your body needs these forces for resisting the diabolic undercurrent of factors that are causing your disease, and for providing the healing energies required to bring your body once more into a state of balance.

 You are faced with a condition that requires all of your resourcefulness, determination, and sense of responsibility toward yourself. It is the greatest challenge to your body's healing abilities, for they cannot work well when overloaded with discouragement and fear. The information in this book is offered as a source of hope. It is extremely realistic to replace hopelessness and negative beliefs with positive possibilities.

The causes of cancer in each patient are different combinations of influences

It is never just one factor
The key to knowing cancer is to recognize it as a multitude of processes working together to destroy your body. Cancer is like a number of diseases attacking your body at the same time. By envisioning the total combination of factors involved in this "attack," you open a new door to understanding cancer, how to manage it, and how to restore your health.

Understanding the nature of cancer
It is no longer justifiable to treat the body as if it were only a mechanical device or system of abnormal cell structures (tumors), while ignoring the connections and influences of the mind to the body, as has been the focus of conventional medicine for the last 100 years.

CANCER is a deterioration of the body, brought about by:

1. Failure of the body cells to obtain all the building materials essential for cell construction and for effective functioning of their structures.
   - » The structural materials of all cells are proteins, minerals, and trace minerals.
   - » All cell functions are performed by enzymes, aided and supported by specific vitamins, minerals, trace minerals, proteins and oils. Without all these working together as a team, cells function poorly, or burn themselves out in the process of trying to function.
   - » All cell and body organs require fuel and energies in order to function. These are oxygen, sugars, special nutrients and life forces.

2. Excess toxicities affect and eventually destroy cells or transform them into abnormal, wild-growing cells known as cancer tumors. These can be and usually are:
   - » Body and cell breakdown products, wastes, toxins, and debris.
   - » Faulty detoxification of and prolonged retention of intestinal wastes.
   - » Environmental, industrial and home chemicals.
   - » Parasites and infections that chronically drain our resources that resist disease.

The most common of environmental hazards and causes of cancer are:

- Chemicals, drugs, poisons, cigarettes, and alcohol.
- Chemical fertilizers, sprays, and pesticides.
- Aerosols, poisonous gases and hydrocarbon fumes.
- Chemical food additives and preservatives.
- Denatured and overcooked foods.
- Dead, devitalized, fast/junk food.
- Pollutants of civilization.

One of the major challenges in trying to identify the cause of cancer is that there is no single culprit and a multitude of possibilities.

3. **Predisposing causes:** Heredity, lifestyle, beliefs, attitudes, behaviors, habits and excesses.

4. **Contributing causes:** Factors creating an environment that is detrimental to cells and favors their eventual degeneration, breakdown and mutation into abnormal cells.

5. **Triggering causes:** Chemicals, trauma, stresses, or environmental abnormalities that overload cells and "break their back" (such as a death of a beloved spouse); factors or forces that weaken the cells' resistance to the onslaught of carcinogens, allowing these poisons to denature and destroy cells.

6. **Carcinogens:** Highly toxic and destructive substances or forces that react directly with the chromosomes of cells, changing their structure in such a way that the control process of cells dividing and multiplying is destroyed. This creates anarchic, wild-growing and abnormal cells that no longer can defend themselves against all the body toxins, wastes and chemicals. The cells absorb these toxic substances. As their growth reaches a certain volume, they start multiplying and dividing at a much more rapid than normal rate and develop into tumors.

   Examples of causal factors that would trigger this process are exposure to: 1) radiation and radon, 2) pesticides, and 3) highly toxic chemicals, dioxins and asbestos.

Contributing Causes of Cancer:
- Failure to live by the laws of nature.
- Neglect of our emotional, mental and physical needs.
- Compromise of our dreams, aspirations, and life purpose.
- Negative attitudes, anxieties, worries, angers, fears, and hatreds.
- Faulty lifestyles; work, play, and habit excesses.
- Faulty reactions to stresses and environmental hazards; overwhelming stresses can set the stage for the onset of cancer. The disease may be induced by feelings of desperation and helplessness or a sense of being out of control. A body that is in a constant state of fight/flight response runs a high risk of exhausting its own immune system.
- Denial of self, of one's self image and true nature; sacrificing self and giving up one's life for another person.
- Overwhelming personal loss.
- Relationships that have been threatening to oneself and one's self-image.
- Emotional relationships that brought pain and doom.
- Negative attitudes, thoughts, beliefs, behaviors & outlooks.

Causes that trigger the flare-up of cancer:
Rarely do cells break down and become transformed into cancer cells unless several different types of causes are interacting and working together. All of these causes drain the body's resources and resistance to disease.

The most important and usually most neglected causes are the multitude of abnormal chemicals that destroy normal cell structures and functions. Before considering and suggesting any practical approaches to dealing with and managing cancer, it is essential to understand the following:

- Our bodies contain poisons, toxins, wastes and pollutants.

- Side effects of conventional allopathic medical treatments—surgery, chemotherapy or radiation—are intensely stressful.

- Smoking alone is not a sufficient explanation for the occurrence of cancer.

    However, a combination of life stress and smoking constitutes a powerful instigator.

Understanding toxins and body poisons – checklist:

- ☐ What are toxins, poisons, body wastes?

- ☐ How do toxins and poisons accumulate and build up hazardous residues?

- ☐ How do our bodies handle and eliminate toxins and body poisons?

- ☐ Cautions we need to take when detoxifying too rapidly.

- ☐ What is the nature of pain?

- ☐ What is the nature of healing? How bodies heal.

- ☐ What are the roles of emotions and lifestyle regarding cancer and cancer healing?

- ☐ What are the many ways we can support and strengthen our body's healing rowers and resistance to cancer? Diet & exercise programs.

- ☐ What hazards, influences or forces block cancer remedies from working?

- ☐ What general counsels can add greatly to the body's self-restoring powers and its resistance to cancer?

Toxins include all substances that are abnormal to, incompatible with, or in excess of the body's needs. These toxins have some form of detrimental effect on cells, organs, and body fluids, or on the balance of body energies and biochemicals. They overload the body, deplete its enzymes and cause systemic fatigue.

Many toxins are manufactured and harbored in our bodies:

- Waste products of cells and organs.

- Mental and emotional toxins; toxins from negative attitudes, hatred, anger, fear, and grief.

- Stress toxins; those that arise in our body from our negative reactions to stress, anxieties, worries, and antagonisms.

Added to these toxins are those that surround, pollute and saturate our environment, providing us with the most chemically hazardous era the world has ever known.

Today it is impossible to breathe air, drink water or eat food without absorbing toxic chemicals and hazardous pollutants.

These toxic substances come under three main categories:
1. Drugs, chemicals, pollutants, and food additives.
2. Processed, overcooked, dead, and unnatural foods, food excesses.
3. Undigested or poorly digested foods.

Thousands of additives, preservatives, colorings, thickeners, sweeteners, pesticides, and chemicals have been insidiously added to or combined with almost all commercial foods. Hundreds of highly toxic chemical wastes, including chlorine, fluoride, chemical fertilizers and industrial wastes, contaminate and denature our drinking waters, food, and the air we breathe.

Many of these pollutants have been proven to cause severe degenerative diseases, including cancer. A large number of pollutants have never been tested to determine their effects on our bodies and on cell functions. We still know little about the dangers to health and the hazards of substances created in the body when various pollutants, chemicals, toxins and/or drugs meet and combine.

In addition to environmental poisons, in the last hundred years our daily diet has changed radically and now includes stale, devitalized, decaying, pressure cooked, over-cooked, microwave-cooked, canned food; food fried to death; and boiled, mummified and dead foods.

We poison ourselves unconsciously, insidiously, constantly and daily. Adding insult to injury, we prolong the stagnation and retention of foods and rotting remnants of foods, year after year, due to constipation and inadequate elimination of body wastes and toxins. The toxic super saturation of our body increases each day we eliminate less than the amount we've eaten.

Each of the billion cells that die every day is a toxin that is the equivalent of a micro-cadaver, a rotting carcass. To some degree, we are poisoning ourselves every single minute of the day. Accept that your body, as healthy as it feels, is miraculously surviving poisons.

Unless you detoxify and eliminate daily, there is no way you can escape the end effects of toxins. It can take up to two years to detoxify the body of a person living in the extreme, abnormal, ecologically dangerous conditions of our civilization.

Consequences of toxic build-up
We have been taught very little about body poisons and have minimal awareness of

exactly how much poison our body is storing. The amounts of toxins, wastes and cell debris that have stagnated and accumulated in our bodies over the years are beyond our normal abilities to appreciate or understand. Nor are we conscious of the great impact of these poisons throughout our entire body. The mere fact that we may be one of those who has a serious disease means that our body is undergoing excessive toxicity saturation.

No one ever realizes the impact of toxins on their body until they have followed an intense detoxifying regime, experienced the initial discomforts and reactions that follow detoxification, and the resulting increase in the wonderful sense of well-being. Without this experience, it is impossible to realize how long it takes to detoxify, or how good one can feel afterward.

Cancer Pain

Body poisons account for 95% of all pain. Only about 5% is triggered by pressures or swelling on the nerves by accidents, blows, and even an increase of blood flow into the area of the pain. Almost all the pain from cancer is created by action on and irritation of nerve endings by body and environmental toxic poisons.

Pain is not a disease. It is not an evil or wrong condition, but rather *the result of a wrong condition*. It is a symptom, a red flag indicating something is wrong, i.e., that a condition exists that needs to be addressed and cared for.

Therefore, the causes of the pain—not the pain itself—should be treated. Use pain killers only in an emergency or when the pain is so intolerable, you are unable to care for yourself in other ways.

Radical detoxification can relieve up to 95% of the pain—even pain that cannot be alleviated by powerful pain-killers such as morphine.

Detoxification

Any good health-restoring regime will release a flood of toxins into the blood and body fluids. Toxic substances are transported by the blood directly to the liver. The liver is the organ equipped to neutralize, detoxify, render harmless and eliminate most body poisons. As long as the liver is healthy and fulfilling its multitude of tasks, healing can progress normally. Essential as support to this liver function are the actions of the other organs of detoxification: colon, kidneys, lungs, skin, and the lymphatic system.

During healing, the body has to rid itself of those poisons that are causing its breakdown. Little or no healing takes place until all toxic and harmful substances are thoroughly eliminated. Any reaction to toxins is an indication that actions must be taken to eliminate them as quickly as possible. Since most of this is done by the liver, it is essential to give your liver every opportunity to perform this task. Liver support should constitute a prime consideration in your healing.

Detoxifying Precautions

It is possible to heal too rapidly by eliminating too many toxins at one time. Going on prolonged fasts or taking large amounts of detoxifying remedies can free the body's stored poisons too quickly. This toxic overload can cause the liver to swell. It is like garbage "plugging up a sponge."

The toxins can saturate and exhaust the liver and organs of detoxification and elimination. This excessive detoxification will leave you feeling as if your treatment is reacting adversely. In fact, you may feel and fear that your treatment is causing harm, which is not really the case. Your body is merely ridding itself of toxins at a rate faster than your organs of detoxification and elimination can keep up with it. During such times, you may experience a toxic "hangover." This is a normal process, similar to the body ridding itself of alcohol after a horrible binge.

At the first sensing of pain, detoxify. Take several enemas. Take them often enough to completely eliminate the poisons causing the pain. Keep taking them until all pain is gone. Take 5, 10, even 15 enemas—whatever number will finally bring you relief.

To avoid or control these unpleasant times of healing, slow down. Give your body time to catch up with the overload. Give it time to break down and eliminate its excess body garbage. Serious and first time toxic reactions can sometimes last weeks. Most "healing crises" normally last four to five days. Your body and its detoxifying organs periodically need a rest. Modify your healing program.

Follow the following recommendations:

- Give your body a two or three day "Sabbath" from your healing regime during the "hangover, healing-crisis"-type reactions. This includes taking a rest from the supplements recommended for healing and rebuilding the body and its immunity.

- *Focus instead on detoxifying.* Increase by doubling or even tripling the amount of supplements that activate and support the organs of detoxification and elimination.

- Throughout the time you are following a therapy, even if you feel comfortable, for one day each week refrain from taking the supplements and remedies in your therapy program that are indicated as healers. Periodically take a weekly healing Sabbath.

- If you feel less well on the days that certain remedies are put aside and you experience some discomfort or let-down, go back on your supplements

Cancer Therapy

You listen to the constant bombardment of threats from doctors who promise you death if you don't undergo chemotherapy, radiation or surgery, "and do it NOW—not next week"—yet they still refuse to promise you success even by following their protocol. You can only get the impression that nothing else can be done for you, i.e., that there are no cures. You are told this every year when cancer fund drives attempt to solicit your checks.

Curing is not finding a doctor who will cure us, but rather finding the "self" we have lost. The first therapy is to eliminate all the causes of cancer—all the multiple, severe abnormalities in our lives, minds, emotions, habits and environment. *We must not expect benefits from any therapy unless we take care of this form of detoxification first.*

To understand and treat any disease, especially cancer, the causes must first be eliminated. If we want to eliminate smoke, we must first quell the flame. This means that we need to determine the causes and also the nature of the cancer.

Hopefully the following section of this book will assure you that *something can be done to help you without destroying much of your health,* as with chemotherapy, radiation and surgery.

The list is practically endless for ways to help you rebuild your health. The key is selecting the therapies that will be most beneficial and effective for your individual health challenge.

Chapter 23

Diet, Cancer & Healing

There are no "incurable" diseases.
There are multitudes of incurable people.

Diet recommendations must be conducive to healing and to satisfying your body needs, completely and precisely. Even foods that may be good for another person with the same disease may not be the best ones for your body requirements.

Cancer is, among other things, a multiple, long term specific enzyme deficiency disease. Enzymes are a most essential and effective part of any cancer therapy. Without the following precautions, dietary restrictions and health measures, healing may not take place.

FOODS THAT FORM THE BASIS OF A CANCER DIET

The foods listed here enhance host resistance and healing. Use as many of these foods as possible, daily and generously.

VEGETABLES

- *Asparagus* - Rich in vitamins A, B-1, B-2, B-3, C; calcium; phosphorus; potassium; iron. Stimulates production of interferon.

- *Cabbage/cabbage juice* - Rich in Vitamin U and fibers; has anti-cancer properties.

- *Celery* - Rich in fiber, enhances immunity and resistance to diseases, flushes kidneys.

- *Carrots* - Rich in Vitamin A, beta-carotene and fiber.

- *Cucumbers* - Rich in potassium and iron; a detoxifier that flushes gall bladder, liver and kidneys.

- *Endive* - Rich in potassium, alkaline minerals and chlorophyll; stimulates saliva and saliva activity; helps cleanse (detoxify) the liver.

- *Spinach* - Rich in Laetrile, chlorophyll and alkalizing minerals.

JUICES
- **Apple** - Vitamin C, potassium.
- **Comfrey** - Chlorophyll, magnesium.
- **Beet**- Potassium, zinc.
- **Grape** - Potassium.
- **Papaya** - Digestive enzymes
- **Carrot** - Vitamin A, beta-carotene.

MISCELLANEOUS
- **Grapes** - Rich in potassium; a good alkalizer and body/blood builder; stimulates spleen, liver and digestive enzymes.
- **Kelp** - Rich in potassium, sodium and all trace minerals.

HERBAL TEAS:
- **Esseniac** - Detoxifier, anti-tumor and cell mutation properties.
- **Chamomile** - Lowers tensions, aids digestion.
- **Chaparral** - Active agents against cancer.
- **Cinnamon** - Stimulates the production of interferon.
- **Comfrey** - Powerful healing properties.
- **Ginseng** - Immunity builder.
- **Golden Seal** - Antibiotic and anti-tumor properties.
- **Licorice** - Stimulates the production of interferon.
- **Pau D'arco** - Anti-tumor properties.
- **Peppermint** - Relaxant, aids digestion.

NUTS & SEEDS
Foods in the following list are rich in Laetrile, a vitamin type ingredient that retards tumor growths.
- **Alfalfa sprouts**
- **Peach pits**
- **Wheat Grass**
- **Buckwheat**
- **Apple seeds**
- **All nuts**
- **Almonds**
- **Prune pits**
- **Apricot pits**
- **Fruit seeds**
- **Beans**
- **Flax seed**

CEREALS & THEIR BRANS
- **Wheat Bran** - Fiber, minerals, calcium; aids toxin elimination.
- **Rice Bran** - Vitamin B, minerals, trace minerals, fiber; enhances immunity, resistance to cancer cell growth.
- **Oat Bran** - Fiber, minerals.
- **Barley** - Enhances immunity and disease resistance; flushes kidneys.
- **Brown Rice and Wild Rice**

MISCELLANEOUS

- *Blackstrap molasses* (unsulfured) - Rich in many alkalizing minerals.
- *Brewer's Yeast* - Vitamins B, chromium, magnesium, iron, phosphorus, selenium, nucleic acids (for chromosomes).
- *Garlic* - Trace minerals, vitamins, iron, calcium, silicon; a blood purifier, diuretic; increases urine flow, a kidney tonic; clears urine of mucus, pus, blood cells; helps drain lymphatic system.
- *Yucca Extract (Optimum D-Tox)* - Powerful detoxifier and intestinal cleanser.

It is most important to stress the consumption of undercooked, fresh, living foods. Obtaining life forces from foods is far more essential than using foods as a source of vitamins, minerals, sugars and proteins. It is also important to avoid feeding the body with any foods (or pills, vitamins, and minerals) that are dead, stale or devitalized.

FORBIDDEN CANCER FOODS

- *Meat* - All flesh meats contain high quantity, low quality proteins. "Poor quality" means poor balance and inadequate amounts of certain amino acids. Commercially sold meat after several weeks of hanging, is dead flesh. All flesh meats are acidifying foods that slow healing.

NOTE: An acid state is the key to breaking down cells, but an alkaline state is the cornerstone of healing. Proper digestion of meats requires great amounts of stomach hydrochloric acid. Avoid all red flesh meats, steaks, roasts, etc.

- *Salt* - Sodium retains water in the body and makes it accumulate. One ounce of salt can retain up to 1 lb. of water. Excess water enters into and bloats cells. Cells that have swollen beyond their normal size divide and multiply. This means that water saturation is a factor that triggers the growth and excess division and multiplication of cells. Salt favors tumor growth.
- *Sea salt*, only the crude or unrefined forms (from health stores) in moderate amounts, is acceptable. Its sodium is low in quantity. Instead of salt for flavoring, use powders of kelp, garlic, onions and other herbal spices.
- *Cheeses* - Even quality cheeses contain up to 1 oz. of salt per lb.
- *Wheat and high gluten foods* - Breads, spaghetti, buns, cookies, pies, cakes, desserts, etc.; these contain excessively high amounts of both salt (up to 1 oz. per lb. of food) and gluten.

  Gluten mixed with our body fluids makes glue, just like the glue we used to make as kids when we mixed flour with water. The blood thickens. This decreases the blood flow, depriving cells of oxygen. Oxygen deprivation is a major problem in cancer.

- **Breads, pastries** - These are inevitably devitalized when cooked or baked (as they usually are) at high temperatures for considerable periods of time. All excess heat destroys essential nutrients. Sprouted wheat breads are acceptable and are best when salt-free. Homemade, salt-free breads of other grains (rye, oats, millet, etc.) are acceptable. Preferable to breads are muffins, for they are cooked for 10 minutes or less.

- **Eggs** - When fresh from naturally fed, range roaming, healthy chickens, eggs could be listed as ideal, balanced foods and an excellent source of most nutrients. These healthy eggs could be a real asset for restoration in most degenerative conditions. However, part of the egg's nutritional value is in its sulphur content. Sulphur favors cell growth, so whenever tumors are present and active it is important to leave eggs out of the diet.

NOTE: Healthy eggs contain lecithin. Lecithin lowers cholesterol.

- **Milk & milk products** - (Exception is unsalted butter) All milk contains excessively high levels of pituitary hormones. These are growth hormones; they promote cell multiplication and tumor growth. Drinking milk eventually depletes hydrochloric acid secretion of the stomach. Pasteurizing milk makes it totally unacceptable as a food for *anyone*. Up to 95% of nutrient values are destroyed or rendered unavailable to the body when milk is pasteurized.

SPECIAL COUNSELS

Dedication and commitment to following a cancer regime must be as meticulous, intense, constant and careful as possible. It should be as serious as the seriousness of the cancer itself. Only by overcoming the causes of the disease and eliminating the disease toxins can one hope to make it possible for any therapy to be effective and successful.

By adhering to all the body's healing and maintenance needs, one has a great chance of recovery, provided of course that the disease has not progressed beyond physical, mental and emotional abilities to administer self-care. Any neglect of the body's needs or cutting back on the healing regime before healing is complete reduces the chance of once again experiencing optimal well-being.

Just as cancer is a long-term disease, taking years, even generations to explode into existence, its healing requires long term, constant care. Every treatment of a serious disease must be followed carefully for two years. This is the time it takes for the normal cells of our bodies to die and be replaced. No treatment should stop until all cells are replaced by a generation of healthy ones.

Since cancer is a very complex disease of the body, mind and emotions, broad and complex protocols and therapies that cover all three of these human aspects must be an ongoing major part of any therapy for it to be effective. It is not possible to disregard these and expect the disease to disappear.

Cancer is a metabolic process rather than just a tumor. A tumor is only the end result of a breakdown of body and cell biochemistry. It then follows that the main therapies must be constantly directed at these biochemical failures rather than at a tumor.

Since cancer is a result of multiple, long term, specific and serious deficiencies, especially of enzymes, it is most important—in fact, essential—that proper nutritional support is a constant and daily part of any program that offers a chance of eradicating both the cancer process and the cancer tumor.

Carcinogens, poisons and toxic chemicals play the most devastating role in denaturing chromosomes and destroying oncogenes that control cell multiplication. **Therefore, the most important aspect of the entire anti-cancer therapy must be targeted at intense detoxification.**

More poisons must be eliminated daily from the body than the total amount of nutrients entering it. If you have three meals daily and you have less than four bowel movements, then you are not flushing out the residues of toxic matter that have been stored for a long time in your body and in your tumors. You are not catching up with the causes of your disease.

Since body healing processes liberate disease-causing poisons from their tumors and the tissues in which they are stored and pour these back into the bloodstream and body fluids, **those poisons must be broken down, neutralized, and/or detoxified and then eliminated from the body**. If they don't go, you don't cure.

As poisons are eliminated from the body storage areas, the body will react. You will experience ups and downs. These poisons can only be transported from their storage spaces to the organs of elimination by the blood. Once they enter the blood they automatically affect all the organs through which this blood passes.

The first organ to which all blood flows is the brain. This is where the reactions of toxicity are experienced. Toxin-saturated blood will always create disturbances in the brain that are upsetting, to say the least. You may experience sensations like pain, headaches, hangover, fatigue, loss of appetite, nausea, nervousness, irritability, sleeplessness, depression, or just plain "feeling lousy."

When experiencing these discomforts do not panic, worry, rush for a pain reducer, take a tranquillizer, or stop your treatments. If anything, be encouraged to realize that healing is taking place and that your treatment is working. There is reason for you to hope and for your morale to go up—not down, but up.

If, or when you experience set-backs, do not get discouraged.

Do not give in to believing your healing is not working.

Do not quit!

Persist in relieving your body of its toxic overloads.

Communicate with your doctor.

REMEMBER: *There are no "incurable" diseases. There are multitudes of incurable people.*

There are disease conditions which have gone beyond the point of curability. There are people who do not perfectly follow their treatments or adhere to their regimes until healing is complete. Failure to get to the bottom of all causes and body needs, resulting in the body's failure to respond to treatment or return to optimal well-being, prompts doctors and lay people alike to label the disease as "incurable."

The role of healing is in your hands. If you are to successfully take charge of becoming your own healer, then the effectiveness and success of all therapies are your responsibility. You must become as fully informed as possible about the nature of your disease, available options and appropriate protocols for all treatments. You must also have a clear understanding of all effects, side effects and consequences associated with the various approaches to your healing program.

ALWAYS maintain confidence in the healing powers of Mother Nature.
Nature always rewards those who give consideration to her needs. In healing as in life in general, our very nature is to *respond* to the good, the pure and the positive, and *react* to the bad, the impure and the negative.

Chapter 24

Healing Is How We Live Our Life

Stick to the fight when you're hardest hit...
It's when things go wrong that you must not quit.

Your healing powers require a great deal of support and encouragement. Without real understanding of how you can help your body, even the best of your healing abilities and the best of therapies can fail. A good therapy mobilizes all the body's resources in such a way that they do not interfere with the healing processes and only create wellness.

Healing principles
- **Innate tendency toward health:** The body has an inner instinct to restore itself to optimum well-being. It also has the power to intuitively and automatically act on that urge, providing we give it the opportunity and do not allow hindering forces and influences.

- **Internal control of the healing processes:** Self-healing is incredibly powerful when we allow it to take charge. It can influence the capacity of the body to fight cancer and reduce stress.

- If all the necessities of living are returned to the body and all the impediments to healing are discarded—provided the disease has not passed beyond "the point of no return"—actually it becomes impossible to stop the healing process. People can heal in spite of chemotherapy, radiation, pain and drugs.

- **Belief that cancer is curable:** Cancer is not an automatic death sentence. In spite of statistics, there's a good possibility for recovery.

It's not possible to have disease in a healthy body. Our bodies know infinitely more about how to heal than doctors, healing professionals or scientists, eg., those who have been trained to address body treatments and therapies, or who research health and medicine.

Use of body-mind techniques can influence our immune system and healing abilities. Psychosocial aspects are part of the "spontaneous remission" of the disease.

Additional suggested basic body-mind approaches to healing are:

- **Relaxation:** Offsets tensions, stresses and distresses.

- **Education:** Delivers more accurate beliefs about the progress and treatment of the cancer. Anxiety and fear of the disease as well as suspicion of the therapy or therapist are deleterious and a waste of the body's resources.

- **Treatment influencing attitudes:** We can either assist our innate processes or we can hinder them as a result of our belief systems, attitudes and behavior. Believing—being convinced and positive about our therapy—is essential. These mindsets affect healing down to the cell level.

  Let go of the past and live for the moment. Live a day at a time. Let tomorrow come with problems. What will be, will be. Do things that are meaningful, enjoyable and fulfilling.

- **Inner peace:** Is attained in part by letting go of past resentments, obligations, guilt, abuses, hurts, grief and losses that one may carry around consciously or even unconsciously.

- **Frequent repetition of visual and mental imaging:** Is important for programming our healing abilities. Imaging fosters inward focusing. We visualize ourselves with perfectly healthy bodies doing activities that energize and please us. This can markedly:
  » Influence the immune system and reduce stress.
  » Help to construct mental images in which we visualize the cancer cells and tumor growths being attacked by the immune system's white blood cells.
  » Enhance and intensify the specific effectiveness of whatever treatment is used.
  » Minimize and control symptoms, distresses, anxieties, fears, etc.

- **Allow the disease to take care of itself in the context of a healthy lifestyle.**

- **Find an external cause:** A purpose for living that is a means for maintaining or increasing a sense of self-fulfillment. If a person's life has no purpose or meaning, the chances of conquering cancer become markedly lessened. Focusing one's whole being on something outside of oneself helps block self-preoccupation and greatly aids healing.

- **Love oneself enough to declare that "I am worthy of continuing to exist."**

- **A will to live, i.e., a desire and determination to recover:** Without this clear volition, virtually nothing else in a treatment makes sense. The promotion of powerful, positive beliefs and attitudes focused on longevity are crucial. Our beliefs program our minds and bodies regarding the actions they will take for healing or for a breakdown of healing.

We all want to live—or we say we do. But is this "wanting to really live," or is it just "not wanting to suffer"? Do we want to live simply to avoid distress for our loved ones, not give up our joys, just "not want to die," or to avoid the fear of death? Are any of these authentic reasons for living?

Essential Supportive Therapies

Understand causes. How have we fostered our own disease? What has our environment contributed to the breakdown of immunity and health? How have the causes taken over our minds?

Question yourself about your values. Asking "why has life given me this suffering?" can become a turning point, a start for seeing life in its vivid realities. It can be a challenge to renew one's attitudes and outlooks. If the challenge is accepted, one can acquire a new peace of mind.

If we make a decision to look at the positives of our life, this new way of thinking and observing ourselves can quiet the inner turmoil, awaken a sense of still being in control of our destiny, and often spark a renewed resistance to the disease with new healing abilities that for many can overcome the cancer.

Manage your life-style with care and consideration.

Essential aspects are:
- Eliminating bad habits and excesses.
- Reducing perceived stresses; releasing tensions.
- Avoiding work and activity excesses which exhaust our reserve energies.
    - » Cut working hours if they are exhausting.
    - » Develop balance between leisure and play, duty and tedious, onerous jobs. Achievement, duty and selfless giving are not the only principles for guiding our lives.
- Keeping active; filling your life with the joys of living.
- Giving the good things in life your priority.
- Adopting a healthier lifestyle, e.g., exercise.
    - » Perform all exercise, even if only walking, doing yoga, or deep breathing, as enjoyment rather than something you need to do

because it's good for you. Exercise performed with a positive attitude promotes improved blood flow, oxygen intake, digestion and elimination. All of these are crucial in cancer care. Adequate blood flow is critical for mobilizing oxygen and white blood cell to fight the disease.

Obtain the support of others. This reinforces all of the previously mentioned therapies. Attempting to rebuild a life and organize a system of living that is capable of resisting disease is not a task one can easily accomplish alone. It is an even more difficult endeavor when one's physical and inner lives seem to be crumbling.

Engage in catharsis. Dumping—getting rid of every negative, every hindrance to healing, every grief, guilt, anxiety, fear, worry, memory of stressful past experiences, has extremely beneficial effects. Seek counseling until you have peace of mind.

Help others. Listen to their problems. Learn from experiences. Go beyond your self-preoccupation. Above all, do not wallow in self-pity.

Take time to think, reflect, and enjoy.

Continue to live carefully, fulfilling all of your physical, mental and emotional needs for a minimum of two years. It can take this long for the body to rid itself of a lifetime of toxic wastes and to replace sick abnormal cells with healthy living ones.

Rest, relax and sleep. Whenever it is difficult to fall asleep or if your sleep is agitated or restless—if your nerves have been tense, up-tight, frayed or upset by excess stresses and tensions—try going for a brisk, perhaps long walk before bedtime. Or exercise enough to start feeling relaxed to the point of feeling tired. However, do not overexert yourself. You will know when to stop.

Make body massage a part of your program. Massage promotes muscle relaxation, blood flow and a sense of well-being.

Avoid excesses of work, play, activity, and exhaustion. Overwork and forcing yourself physically to the point of exhaustion can block healing. Your body energies should be reserved as much as possible for healing: maintaining abilities to regenerate new cells and tissues and staying on a high level of immunity and resistance to breakdown factors.

Avoid excesses of stresses, distresses and tensions. Obviously this is not always possible or realistic. Whenever your life is overloaded with stresses and problems, these issues create discomforts beyond a reasonable ability to tolerate. During these times it is essential that you enhance your body's abilities to withstand the abuses and excesses. We cannot change certain events in our lives, but we can learn to change the ways we respond to them.

This can be done through the use of specific supplements, such as "Optimum D-Tox," a concentrated yucca extract loaded with an abundance of natural occurring anti-stress compounds.

Remember the two rules in life for dealing with stress:
1. Don't sweat the little stuff
2. It's all small stuff

Live spiritually. When cancer strikes, our faith and beliefs are crucial. Cancer forcefully brings to us an awareness of death, possibly for the first time. All aspects and issues of our existence, including our life purpose, can seem to have lost their meaning. Cancer can influence its victims to review their life in terms of its values and purpose. Any confrontation with potential death can be a great teacher.

Pray. Visualize the afterlife. This can be comforting to those who believe in an afterlife. Returning to the realization that the real purpose of living is what follows our life here takes the sting out of dying. The cancer loses its threat and power over us.

Control and balance your nutrition so that it responds to each of your body's needs.

Healing is far more than mere recovery from bodily diseases and freedom from symptoms. Real recovery and total wellness demand harmony among the physical, spiritual, mental and emotional domains. It is a dynamic state of intense and joyful living, of self-fulfillment and balance.

*"Healing"—being whole and ensuring wholeness—
really is how we live our life!*

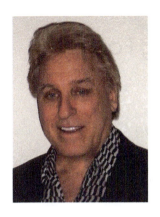

About The Author

Doug Widdifield

For the past 30+ years, Canadian born Doug Widdifield has devoted his energy, skills and expertise to both the development and marketing of organic botanical products—for industrial, agricultural and human consumption.

In the early 1980s, Doug started researching a desert plant known as 'yucca'. Over the next several years he successfully formulated and marketed well over 30 different yucca products. In 1988, Doug turned his attention to studying the human health benefits as a result of his introduction to Dr. Robert Bingham—who at the time, was the foremost authority on arthritis and had completed 'double blind' studies using the same particular yucca species (namely *schidigera* or its more common name 'Mojave yucca').

With Dr. Bingham's inspiration and the assistance of a master herbalist, several renowned doctors, along with the medical science department at the University of Calgary—Doug developed the 'first' liquid nutritional supplement based on the 'schidigera' yucca species.

In 1989, Doug established a Canadian company—to distribute his 'proprietary' schidigera yucca nutritional product for humans. During this time, Doug developed the only western based herbal therapies to receive an unprecedented approval by the Federal Ministry of Health in China—as holistic modalities—and with DIN #s and import permits. He has had the privilege of lecturing throughout China, Hong Kong, South Korea, Singapore, Canada and the U.S. Oftentimes accompanying him were Medical and Naturopathic doctors.

In 2000 Doug sold his company and devoted his time to consulting, lecturing, educating and conducting advanced product research. In 2005 Doug, along with his wife Krystyna (also from Canadian roots) co-founded Zenus LLC—a Nevada Corporation. Doug currently serves as President of Zenus LLC and works closely with Krystyna in developing an exclusive 'Optimum Wellness' product line for humans and animals, all of which strictly adhere to their philosophy of being "complete whole food" nutritional supplements. Zenus' proprietary natural health formulations are now sold in 16 countries and expanding rapidly. Thousands of unsolicited testimonials attest to the amazing healing properties of these amazing 'whole food herbal supplements'—derived from nature.

Says Doug…*"My fabulous wife Krystyna and I live by one motto: We can get everything we want out of life simply by helping others get what they want."* Doug currently teaches a course on Health & Wellness at UNLV in Las Vegas, NV and resides with his wife in Henderson, NV.

Appendix

Chart of Acid- & Alkaline-Forming Foods*

CODE (1) Fresh picked, neutral
(after 24 hours from stalk they become increasingly acid.)

The following is a list foods which are acid-forming and also foods which are alkaline-forming.

The comparative qualities of the various foods in the list are indicated by X's
> 1 X = mild, low excises of acid or alkaline
> 2 X's = moderate levels of acid or alkaline
> 3 X's = strong, high levels
> 4 X's = very strong acidity/alkalinity, very high levels.

* *Acid means acidifying; some alkaline foods are acidifying. (proteins). Alkaline means alkalizing; some acid foods are alkalizing (fruits).*

COMPARATIVE ACIDITY AND ALKALINITY OF FOODS

Recommended Quality Foods	Acid	Alkaline
Almonds, unsalted		X
Apples, fresh		XX
Apples, dried		XX
Apricots, fresh		XXX
Apricots, dried		XXXX
Asparagus		XX
Bananas, ripe	XX	
Barley	X	
Beans, Navy, baked	XXX	
Beans, green, fresh in pods		XXX
Beef	XX	
Beets, fresh		XXX
Berries, all kinds .		XX to XXXX
Cabbage		XXX
Cantaloupe		XXX
Carrots		XXXX
Cauliflower		XXX
Celery		XXXX
Chard		XXX
Cheese, hard, aged	XX	
Cherries		XX
Chicken	XXX	
Corn, dried		X
Cranberries	X to XX	
Currants	XXX	

Recommended Quality Foods	Acid	Alkaline
Cucumbers, fresh		XXXX
Dandelion, greens		XXX
Dates		XX
Eggs, whole	XXX	
Eggs, whites	XXXX	
Figs, dried		XXXX
Fish	XX to XXX	
Fruits, nearly all		XXX
Game meat	XX to XXX	
Halibut steak	XXX	
Lamb	XXX	
Lamb stew	X	
Lemon juice, natural		XXX
Lettuce		XXXX
Lima Beans, fresh		XXX
Lima Beans, dry	X	
Liver beef	XXX	
Muskmelon, *alone		XXX
Mutton	XX	
Oatmeal, cooked	XXX	
Oils, from seeds, grains, nuts	XX – XXX	
Onions		XX
Orange juice, natural		XXX
Parsnips		XXX
Peaches		XXX
Peanuts	XX	
Pears		XX
Pecans	XX	
Peppers		XXX
Plums	XX	
Peas, fresh, green		X
Peas ripe, dry	XX	
Pineapple		XXX
Potatoes, white		XXX
Potatoes, sweet (6)	X to ?	
Prune	XX – XXX	
Pumpkins		X
Radishes		XXX
Raisins		XX
Rhubarb		XXX
Rye, other seed grains	XX – XXX	
Salmon	XXX	
Spinach		XXXX
Squash, summer		XX
Squash, winter	X	
Tomatoes, fresh		XXXX
Tomatoes, canned		XXX
Turkey	XX	
Turnips		XX
Walnuts	X	
Watermelons		XXX

* melon should always be eaten alone, not mixed with other fruit.

Poor Quality, NOT Recommended Faulty Foods	Acid	Alkaline
Bacon, fat	X	
Bacon, lean	XX	
Bread, white, milk	XX	
Bread, wheat / whole grains	X	
Cheese, cottage	X	
Clams	XXX	
Corn flour	XX	
Cornstarch	X	
Fruits, stewed, sugared	X to XXX	
Grape juice, sweetened	XXX	
Lobsters, Crabs	XXXX	
Olives, ripe, dried		XXX
Olives, green, pickled	XX	
Oysters	XXXX	
Pork, lean	XX	
Rice, natural/polished	XX	
Shredded Wheat	XX	
Veal	XXX	
Wheat, whole, cracked	XX	

Recommended Products:

I personally use and endorse all dietary supplements from Zenus LLC
ZenusGlobalHealth.com
—who manufacture *only* **'complete whole food'** supplements.

- OPTIMUM D-TOX (whole food extract from the Mojave yucca)

- ESSENIAC HERBAL TEA (original Native Ojibway formula)

- POWRE (proprietary watermelon rind extract)

- C-FOOD (highest source of complete vitamin C)

- KELATE (synergistic complete food source for eliminating heavy toxic metals)

Recommended Reading:

"THE UNIVERSAL LAWS OF HEALING"
(The Contrast Between Healers And Pretenders)
by Dr. C.C. Wilcher, D.C., N.D.

"YOUR HEALTH IS YOUR CHOICE"
(Health Made Simple)
by Dennis Richard

For information on speaking engagements, lectures, seminars etc.
contact me—Doug Widdifield at dougwiddifield@gmail.com

'Be careful about reading health books.
You may die of a misprint.'
— Mark Twain

CPSIA information can be obtained at www.ICGtesting.com
Printed in the USA
BVOW10s0135120913

330989BV00001B/1/P